Handbook of Heart Transplantation

Handbook of
Heart Transplantation

Edited by Calvin White

hayle
medical

New York

Hayle Medical,
750 Third Avenue, 9th Floor,
New York, NY 10017, USA

Visit us on the World Wide Web at:
www.haylemedical.com

ISBN: 978-1-63241-561-5

Cataloging-in-Publication Data

Handbook of heart transplantation / edited by Calvin White.
    p. cm.
Includes bibliographical references and index.
ISBN 978-1-63241-561-5
1. Heart--Transplantation. 2. Heart--Surgery. 3. Heart--Diseases.
4. Cardiology. I. White, Calvin.
RD598.35.T7 H36 2019
617.412 059 2--dc23

Table of Contents

Preface

This book was inspired by the evolution of our times; to answer the curiosity of inquisitive minds. Many developments have occurred across the globe in the recent past which has transformed the progress in the field.

A heart transplant is a surgical transplantation procedure that is performed on patients suffering from severe coronary artery disease or end-stage heart failure. A functioning heart from a recently deceased organ donor is implanted into a patient when other medical or surgical treatments have failed to suffice. It is not considered a cure but a life-saving treatment that is intended to improve the chances of survival and provide a better quality of life to individuals. Patients who do not qualify for a heart transplant may be prescribed a left ventricular assist device (LVAD) or an artificial heart. In some cases, a heart-lung transplant is performed in patients with diseased heart and lungs. Nearly 3,500 heart transplant surgeries are performed worldwide every year. The survival period post-operation is averaged to be at 15 years. This book presents the complex aspects of heart transplantation in the most comprehensible and easy to understand language. Different approaches, evaluations, methodologies and advanced studies on heart transplantation have been included in this book. It will be a valuable resource for cardiologists, cardiac surgeons, residents and students alike.

This book was developed from a mere concept to drafts to chapters and finally compiled together as a complete text to benefit the readers across all nations. To ensure the quality of the content we instilled two significant steps in our procedure. The first was to appoint an editorial team that would verify the data and statistics provided in the book and also select the most appropriate and valuable contributions from the plentiful contributions we received from authors worldwide. The next step was to appoint an expert of the topic as the Editor-in-Chief, who would head the project and finally make the necessary amendments and modifications to make the text reader-friendly. I was then commissioned to examine all the material to present the topics in the most comprehensible and productive format.

I would like to take this opportunity to thank all the contributing authors who were supportive enough to contribute their time and knowledge to this project. I also wish to convey my regards to my family who have been extremely supportive during the entire project.

Editor

Heterotopic Heart Transplantation

Hannah Copeland and Jack G. Copeland

Abstract

The heterotopic heart transplant was pioneered by Christian Barnard in the late 1970s as a way to treat acute rejection in the pre-cyclosporine era. The technique was also used for the treatment of severe pulmonary hypertension, in patients unable to have an orthotopic heart transplant. Some surgeons have used the heterotopic heart transplant as a way to increase the donor heart pool around the world in more recent years. The heterotopic heart transplant is a good viable option for severe pulmonary hypertension patients, and, severe pulmonary vascular resistance patients, who would otherwise, not qualify for an orthotopic heart transplant. The outcomes for these recipients have been comparable to survival outcomes for similar orthotopic heart transplant recipients.

Keywords: heterotopic, transplant, heart

1. Introduction

By August of 1975 [1], 277 patients had received an orthotopic heart transplantation and 49 were alive. The longest survivor lived 6.8 years.

Christian Barnard reported the heterotopic heart transplant (HHT) technique. In 1976 [1], Barnard noted the benefits of heterotopic heart transplantation to be that the donor heart acts as an assist device, assists during episodes of rejection, can be removed in case of severe graft rejection, and still the patient may receive a subsequent heart transplant. Barnard et al. [2] published a case report of a heterotopic heart transplant recipient that suffered acute rejection and was supported by the native heart while the heterotopic graft recovered.

At the time the paper was written, cyclosporine was not used for post-heart transplantation and the incidence of acute rejection was more common. The heterotopic heart transplant technique offered an extra layer of prevention and/or treatment during the pre-cyclosporine era when death within 24 hours of the onset of rejection was common. In addition, to the benefits from treatment of acute rejection, the heterotopic heart transplantation technique allows selected recipients with pulmonary hypertension to receive a transplant.

2. Heterotopic heart transplantation history and current use

Between 1974 and 1982, Barnard performed 40 heterotopic heart transplants [3]. The first year, second year and five-year survival for heterotopic heart transplantation was 61, 50 and 36%. These survival rates compared well to the orthotopic heart transplant survival from Stanford of 63% at 1 year, 55% at 2 years and 39% at 5 years. The Copeland group from the University of Arizona, during the same time demonstrated 72% 1 and 2-year survival with orthotopic heart transplantation [3].

Bleasdale et al. [4] published the use of 42 consecutive, adult heterotopic heart transplantations in a single center from 1993 to 1999 and compared the outcomes to 303 consecutive orthotopic heart transplants (OHT) during the same time period. Thirty-three (33; 79%) of the heterotopic heart transplant recipients were men; and 26 recipients had ischemic heart disease (62%). In the comparative group of orthotopic heart transplant recipients, 38% had ischemic heart disease and 43% were dilated cardiomyopathy patients. The reasons for using a HHT in these recipients was urgency and need for transplant (36%), pulmonary hypertension of the recipient (55%), donor-recipient size mismatch [donor body surface area (BSA) < 75% of the recipient BSA] (62%); and the native heart was able to be repaired (19%). The patients were followed from 1 to 5 years. The heterotopic heart transplant recipients were older, more often had a donor-recipient size mismatch, and had a higher ischemic time. The ischemic time the HHT group was on average 191 minutes (165–241 minutes) vs. 165 minutes (120–202 minutes) in the orthotopic heart transplant group; which was statistically significant (p = 0.001). The OHT group had a higher 30-day survival of 87 vs. 76% HHT group. The 1-year survival was higher for the OHT group 74 vs. 59%. The three factors that predicted graft failure were: (1) donor recipient size mismatch, (2) donor age, and, (3) the female donor. The donors in the HHT group more often had a size mismatch, were older, and female. Of note, within the HHT group, those who were size matched had a markedly improved 1-year survival 81 vs. 45% (p = 0.02).

Overall, in the Bleasdale et al. [4] study HHT recipients had decreased 1-year survival. The decreased survival was predominantly in patients who had received a donor-recipient mismatched heart. The survival for size matched was comparable to those patients who received an orthotopic heart transplant. In addition, patients with severe and/or fixed pulmonary hypertension benefitted from the HHT; when, these recipients would not have been able to have an OHT.

Newcomb et al. [5] described the use of the heterotopic heart transplant to expand the donor pool in Australia. During a 6-year period from 1997 to 2003, the group performed 20 heterotopic heart transplants and 131 orthotopic heart transplants. The heterotopic heart transplant was used for: (1) fixed pulmonary hypertension (with a pulmonary vascular resistance greater than or equal to 3 Wood units, and a transpulmonary gradient (TPG) greater than or equal to 13 mmHg), (2) donor to recipient weight ratio of less than 0.8, (3) anticipated ischemic time greater than 6 hours, and (4) a marginal donor heart. Marginal donors were described as those that required high inotropic support, had a history of a cardiac arrest or arrhythmia, wall motion abnormalities on the echocardiogram, and/or ischemic changes on the electrocardiogram (EKG). Fourteen of the donor hearts were marginal and had been declined by other centers. Most of the HHT recipients had more than one indication for an HHT.

In the study of Newcomb et al. [5], the heterotopic heart transplant recipients were significantly older (mean 58 years vs. 47.1 years for OHT); the donors were also significantly older (mean age 45.2 years vs. 34.5 years for OHT). The ischemic time was also much higher for the HHT recipients; 366 minutes vs. 258 minutes for OHT. The intensive care unit and the total length of the hospital stay was higher for HHT recipients; though, not statistically significant. The study demonstrated lower survival for heterotopic heart transplant recipients compared to orthotopic heart transplant recipients in the same time period; though, the survival benefit for OHT recipients disappeared when they performed a subgroup analysis for the recipients who had elevated pulmonary artery pressures. The study demonstrates the successful use of the heterotopic heart transplant. The survival in HHT recipients were not as good as in those of OHT recipients because of the HHT technique was more often used in marginal donors and more high-risk recipients. Marginal donor hearts may not have performed as well in OHT recipients. Furthermore, high risk recipients have decreased survival expectations especially with the use of a marginal donor heart.

Boffini et al. [6] described their single center experience with the heterotopic heart transplant; and, found the HHT to be comparable to OHT. HHT was used between in 1985–2003, in 12 patients [(1.7%) of the all the heart transplant performed during that time]. The 1-year and 5-year survival was 92 and 64% respectively. These results demonstrated when the HHT technique is used in the usual recipient risk patient, the outcomes can be effective and acceptable for recipients. The HHT technique was used for body size mismatch in 11 patients and 1 recipients for a marginal donor heart.

In addition to donor-recipient size mismatch, elevated pulmonary vascular resistance (PVR), and, fixed pulmonary hypertension are also indications for HHT. Vassileva et al. [7] reviewed 18 recipients with fixed pulmonary vascular resistance who received a HHT with the donor pulmonary artery anastomosed to the recipient right atrium. The indications were (1) PVR > 6 units/m^2, (2) transpulmonary gradient (TPG) > 15 mmHg, or, (3) pulmonary artery (PA) systolic pressure > 60 mmHg. All of the recipients had some degree of pulmonary hypertension, and, 8 of the patients had a restrictive cardiomyopathy. Twelve of the patients were New York Heart Association class III or IV; the remaining six were in the hospital with continuous inotropic support, and, one was intubated. The mean aortic cross clamp time was 58 minutes and a mean ischemic time of 122 minutes. The follow-up right heart catheterizations demonstrated a progressive decrease in the pulmonary artery pressures after transplant with a mean systolic pulmonary artery pressure of 29 mmHg, a TPG of 10 mmHg, and, a PVR of 3.7 units/m^2. The group concluded that the HHT technique was a valuable option for patients with elevated, and/or, fixed pulmonary artery pressures, and, elevated pulmonary vascular resistance.

3. The heterotopic surgical technique

There are two published surgical techniques for the heterotopic heart transplant. Novitzky et al. [8] published the first surgical technique pioneered by Christian Barnard in the 1970s. The heterotopic transplant technique pioneered by Barnard started with the anastomosis of the donor left atrium to the recipient left atrium. Then, the donor right atrium is anastomosed to the recipient right atrium and superior vena cava. Next, the donor aorta is sutured to the recipient aorta in an end to side fashion. The pulmonary anastomosis is the remaining anastomosis. The pulmonary artery is sutured to a dacron graft. The dacron graft is used to extend the anastomosis to the recipient pulmonary artery. Without the interposition graft, the donor and recipient pulmonary arteries would not be able to be brought together without tension or possibly not at all because of lack of length on the donor tissue (**Figure 1**).

In 2017, Copeland et al. [9] published an alternate heterotopic heart transplant technique as a biologic left ventricular assist. The donor heart left pulmonary veins and inferior vena cava are oversewn. The right pleura is widely opened, and the right posterior pericardium is opened toward the phrenic nerve at the level of the diaphragm, cephalad and in-between. The donor and recipient left atria are anastomosed first. Then, the donor aorta is anastomosed to the recipient aorta in an end to side fashion. The aortic cross clamp is removed, and, the patient is placed in Trendelenburg position. The donor pulmonary artery is anastomosed to the recipient right atrium. The donor superior vena cava (SVC) is anastomosed to the recipient superior vena cava in an end to side fashion (**Figure 2**). The anastomosis of the SVC is marked with clips, in order to be able to identify the anastomosis later for endomyocardial biopsy through the right internal jugular vein.

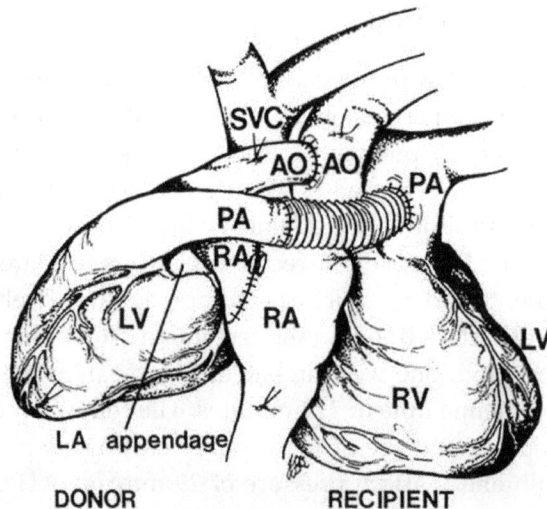

Figure 1. The Barnard heterotopic heart transplant technique with an interposition Dacron Graft. Permission Granted by Annals of Thoracic Surgery for reprint. Novitzky et al. [8].

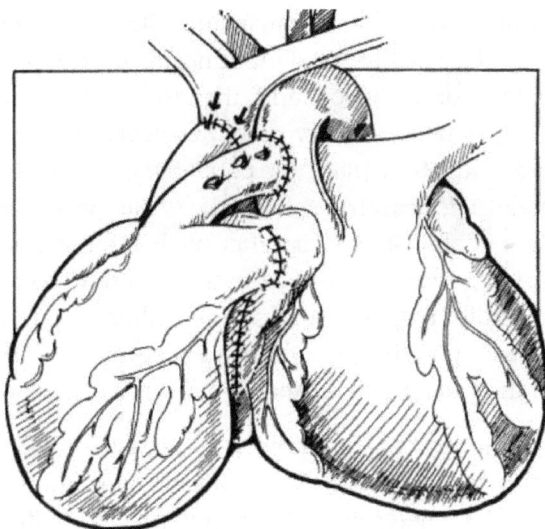

Figure 2. The Copeland heterotopic heart transplant technique. Permission granted by Annals of Thoracic Surgery for reprint. Arzouman et al. [13].

4. Series of patients with heterotopic heart transplants

The Copeland heterotopic heart transplant technique was used in the series of patients at the University of Arizona and University of California San Diego (by Jack Copeland). Between May 1984 to February 2011, 5 patients received a heterotopic heart transplant. The reasons for a heterotopic heart transplantation included the following: (1) fixed pulmonary hypertension with pulmonary artery (PA) pressures of 85/53 mmHg with a mean of 60 mmHg and pulmonary vascular resistance of 10 Woods units, (2) severe pulmonary hypertension of 85/30 mmHg with a mean of 48 mmHg and a PVR of 6 Woods units, (3) PA pressure of 69/34 mmHg with a trans-pulmonary artery gradient of 17 mmHg and pulmonary vascular resistance of 9 Woods units, and (4) and (5) donor recipient size mismatch in two patients.

Of the three patients with severe pulmonary hypertension, one was a 9-year old child was diagnosed with restrictive cardiomyopathy and had heart failure since early infancy [10]. The patient presented for transplant evaluation with incessant supraventricular tachycardia and pulmonary hypertension with a PA pressure of 85/53 mmHg with a mean of 60, and, a PVR of 10 Woods units. The patient's cardiac index was 3.1 l/min/sqM with an ejection fraction of 33% on echocardiogram with normal right ventricular function. The fractional shortening on the echocardiogram was 18%. The patient began to develop hepatomegaly and the total bilirubin was elevated to 2.8 mg/dl. The patient was on medical management for heart failure prior to transplant including: furosemide, spironolactone, digoxin, captopril, amiodarone, coumadin and prednisone. The patient was not on inotropic therapy. The patient was listed for heart transplantation and it was deemed that the child would not tolerate an orthotopic heart transplant because of the fixed pulmonary hypertension. The patient was not eligible for a left ventricular assist device (LVAD) because pediatric LVADs were not available in North America until 2000; when the first was implanted in North America.

The patient underwent a heterotopic heart transplant with the Copeland technique [9]. The patient was treated with standard institutional immunosuppressive therapy in 1997; including, rabbit antithymocyte globulin for induction, and, then followed with cyclosporine, mycophenolate and prednisone. The pulmonary artery pressures never decreased throughout the post-transplant course. At 13 years post-transplant, the patient began to have heart failure symptoms, and was re-listed for a heterotopic heart transplant. The patient was status 1B on and died while waiting for heart transplant at almost 14 years after his heterotopic heart transplant. Of note, Al-Khaldi et al. [11] reported a case report of 22-month-old who received a heterotopic heart transplant for restrictive cardiomyopathy and severe pulmonary hypertension. The patient required sildenafil in the post-operative period due to post-operative pulmonary hypertensive crisis, and, with sildenafil the patient was weaned from ventilator support and extubated.

The second patient also had severe pulmonary hypertension of 85/30 with a mean of 48 mmHg, and, a PVR of 6 Woods units. Due to his elevated pulmonary arterial pressure, the patient was listed and had a heterotopic heart transplant. He did not have clinical right heart failure. At one-year post-transplant, the pulmonary artery pressures decreased to 39/18 with a mean of 28 mmHg. Post-transplant, he had one episode of acute rejection that required hospitalizations treated with solumedrol. In addition, he had delirium and psychosis, the steroids were decreased, and the patient improved. The patient lived well for 6 years without complications. He presented to the hospital in respiratory distress. The autopsy demonstrated a pulmonary embolus, with esophageal and gastric ulcerations.

The third patient was a 36-year-old with pulmonary arterial hypertension, a dilated left ventricle with an 15% ejection fraction [a left ventricular end diastolic dimension (LVEDD) of 7.2 cm], and a slightly dilated right ventricle with preserved function and no right heart failure. His PA pressures were 69/34 mmHg with a mean of 47 with a transpulmonary gradient of 17 mmHg and a pulmonary vascular resistance of 9 Woods units. In the face of minimal evidence for right heart failure, a heterotopic heart transplant was performed. He was extubated on the first post-operative day and had normal graft function (LV ejection fraction of 64%), normal exercise tolerance, no right heart failure and a drop in his systolic PA pressure to 48 by trans-thoracic echo. Sadly, he remained impoverished and had great difficulty complying with post transplantation management. Three years later, he died of graft failure most likely from rejection.

The fourth patient was in the intensive care unit (ICU) on multiple inotropes; dobutamine, dopamine, and phenylephrine. A donor heart was accepted. The team knew the donor was "small" (5'5" and 60 kg) compared to the 6'2.5" and 90 kg recipient. The recipient was left awake in the operating room until the donor heart arrived. The surgeon (Jack Copeland) examined the donor heart and found it to be too small for an orthotopic transplant. The option of heterotopic placement was then discussed with the patient with a full explanation of increased risk from the size discrepancy. The recipient agreed to proceed. He survived for 11 months, leading a very active "normal" life. The patient succumbed to a recurrence of alcoholism associated with poor compliance and profound rejection. Prior to his demise, the patient had called the hospital relating symptoms of heart failure but was snowed in and unable to leave his home due to weather conditions. The patient had not taken his immunosuppressive medications for several days.

The fifth patient had a severely dilated left ventricle, with an 8 cm end diastolic dimension. He also was critically ill and was transplanted with a small donor heart (4.5 cm left ventricular end diastolic dimension (LVEDD)]. He survived for 9.5 years. As time passed his LV continued to enlarge and he developed recurrent ventricular tachycardia of the native heart accompanied by chest pain and was treated with high dose amiodarone therapy. The side effects of the amiodarone were significant including bradycardia, lethargy, and exercise intolerance. He also had blue facial discoloration. His cardiac graft function was normal on transesophageal echocardiogram. He refused relisting for orthotopic transplantation. We also offered him a left ventricle cardiectomy of the native heart and he declined. He died at home suddenly 9.5 years post transplantation of unknown causes.

5. Conclusion and discussion

Heterotopic heart transplant patients require endomyocardial biopsies as do orthotopic heart transplant recipients. Barnard first described the endomyocardial biopsy in heterotopic heart transplant patients in 1982. [12] Arouzman et al. [13] also described the use of the endomyocardial biopsy in conjunction with the Copeland heterotopic heart transplant technique [9] by leaving clips at the SVC anastomosis for visualization at the time of endomyocardial biopsy (**Figure 3**).

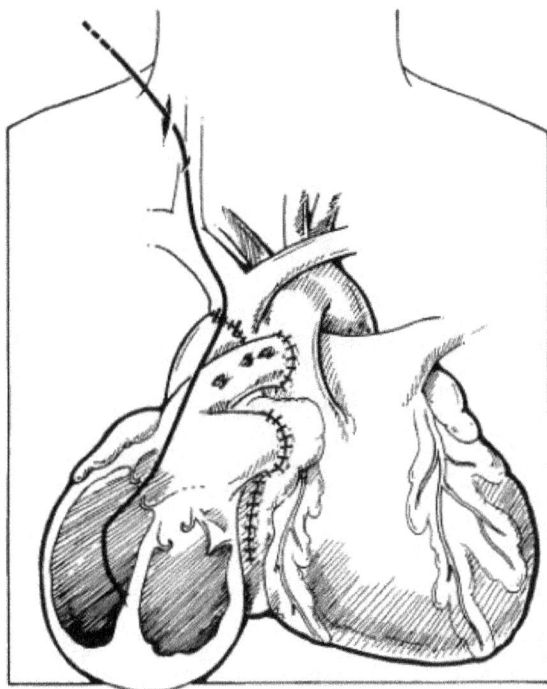

Figure 3. Endomycardial biopsy of the donor heart in a heterotopic heart transplant. Permission granted by Annals of Thoracic Surgery for reprint. Arzouman DA et al. [13].

Heterotopic heart transplantation is a valuable treatment option for patients with severe and/ or fixed pulmonary hypertension and severe pulmonary vascular resistance in the absence of native right ventricular failure. The patient cannot have an orthotopic heart transplant. Even though they may benefit from mechanical circulatory support, these patients would still benefit from a heterotopic heart transplant. The heterotopic heart transplant recipients described above lived well and had the typical post-heart transplant survival as an orthotopic heart transplant. HHT recipients must be followed as orthotopic heart transplants, have the same immunosuppression regimens and post-transplant biopsy schedule. A heterotopic heart transplant, will allow symptomatic improvement in the recipients with severe pulmonary hypertension and severely elevated PVR. Such patients may forgo LVAD implantation with attendant complications and short-term survival. Some of these patients with HHT may experience reduction of PVR while others may not such as the young heterotopic heart transplant recipient who barely had a decrease in PA pressures over the almost 14-year post-transplant course.

Based on the literature, it is difficult to determine if the heterotopic heart transplant would increase the donor pool by using size mismatched hearts. In the literature, Bleasdale et al. [4], and Newcomb et al. [5], note that the heterotopic heart transplant recipients had decreased survival compared to orthotopic heart transplant recipients. Though, the recipients in those studies were not as good candidates as the orthotopic recipients, and the heterotopic donor hearts were also considered marginal donors, often declined by other centers. Thus, the heterotopic heart transplant may still be a valuable option to increase the donor pool if the donors are not marginal and not used in less than ideal heart transplant recipients. The literature and patient review demonstrates that severe pulmonary hypertension and elevated pulmonary vascular resistance are clear indications for heterotopic heart transplantation with good survival outcomes.

Author details

Hannah Copeland[1*] and Jack G. Copeland[2]

*Address all correspondence to: hannahcopeland411@gmail.com

1 University of Mississippi Medical Center, Jackson, Mississippi, United States of America

2 University of Arizona, Tucson, Arizona, United States of America

References

[1] Barnard CN. Heterotopic versus orthotopic heart transplantation. Transplantation Proceedings. 1976;**8**(1):15-19

[2] Barnard CN, Losman JG, Curcio CA, et al. The advantage of heterotopic cardiac transplantation over orthotopic cardiac transplantation in the management of severe acute rejection. The Journal of Thoracic and Cardiovascular Surgery. 1977 Dec;**74**(6):918-924

[3] Hassoulas J, Barnard CN. Heterotopic cardiac transplantation. SA Medical Journal. 1984 April;**65**:675-682

[4] Bleasdale RA, Banner NR, Anyanwyu AC, et al. Determinants of outcome after heterotopic heart transplantation. The Journal of Heart and Lung Transplantation. 2002;**21**:867-873

[5] Newcomb AE, Esmore DS, Rosenfeldt FL, et al. Heterotopic heart transplantation: An expanding role in the twenty-first century? The Annals of Thoracic Surgery. 2004;**78**: 1345-1351

[6] Boffini M, Ragni T, Pellegrini, et al. Heterotopic heart transplantation: A single-centre experience. Transplantation Proceedings. 2004;**36**:638-640

[7] Vassileva A, Valsecchi O, Sebastiani R, Fontana A, et al. Heterotopic heart transplantation for elevated pulmonary vascular resistance in the current era: Long-term clinical and hemody-namic outcomes. The Journal of Heart and Lung Transplantation. 2013 Sept;**32**(9):934-936

[8] Novitzky D, Cooper DKC, Barnard CN. The surgical technique of heterotopic heart trans-plantation. The Annals of Thoracic Surgery. 1983;**36**:476-482

[9] Copeland J, Copeland H. Heterotopic heart transplantation: Technical considerations. Operative Techniques in Thoracic and Cardiovascular Surgery. 2017;**21**:269-280

[10] Copeland H, Kalra N, Gustafson M, et al. A case of heterotopic heart transplant as a "bio-logic left ventricular assist" in restrictive cardiomyopathy. World Journal of Pediatric and Congenital Heart Surgery. 2011 Oct;**2**(4):637-640

[11] Al-Khaldi A, Reitz BA, Zhu H, et al. Heterotopic heart transplant combined with postoper-ative sildenafil use for the treatment of restrictive cardiomyopathy. The Annals of Thoracic Surgery. 2006;**81**:1505-1507

[12] Cooper DKC, Fraser RC, Rose AG, et al. Technique, complications, and clinical value of endomyocardial biopsy in patients with heterotopic heart transplants. Thorax. 1982;**37**: 727-731

[13] Arzouman DA, Arabia FA, Sethi GK, et al. Endomyocardial biopsy in the heterotopic heart transplant patient. The Annals of Thoracic Surgery. 1998;**65**:857-858

2

Mechanical Circulatory Support as Bridge to Pediatric Heart Transplantation

Martin Schweiger and Michael Huebler

Abstract

Fueled by the uncertainty and the time required to obtain a donor heart, mechanical circulatory support (MCS) forms an essential part of end-stage heart failure. Extracorporeal membrane oxygenation (ECMO) use is limited to a few days before serious complications like bleeding occur. Prolonged support in terms of ventricular assist device (VAD) as a bridge to transplantation (BTT) became mandatory to overcome death on the waiting list. Within the last decade, VADs in adults have evolved drastically with the introduction of continuous flow (cf) devices. Increased miniaturization of VADs and new support strategies have increased its use in the pediatric population even in small children and patients with congenital heart disease (CHD). Nevertheless, patient and device selection in this patient population remain challenging to achieve optimal outcome and decrease complication rates. This comes with the need for care providers specialized in this field. Size issues and anatomical diversity make decision making complex and unique when compared to general adult practice. Neonates with single ventricle physiology are the highest risk candidates for VADs. This chapter reviews the most relevant durable VADs used in children including the rapid evolution of using adult designed cf-VADs to support children with anatomical normal hearts and CHD.

Keywords: pediatric ventricular assist device, pediatric heart transplantation, bridge to transplantation, congenital heart disease, Berlin Heart EXCOR pediatric

1. Introduction

Hospitalization among children suffering from end-stage heart failure (HF) is increasing [1]. If not otherwise correctable and in the absent of contraindications, heart transplantation

(HTx) remains the treatment of choice. Pediatric HTx (pHTx) represents a small but very special part in the field of cardiac transplantation. Children remain at an increased risk of death on the waiting list for HTx [2]; especially infant heart transplant recipients are at a greater risk of death compared to older children. The main reason is the search for an appropriately sized organ donor [2–4]. The limited numbers of available pediatric donor heart organs led to an increased mean waiting time in most Western countries [4]. Tapping all potential brain-dead donors and expanding the recipient pool on an international level is thus of vital importance especially for smaller countries in Europe. Therefore, international organ exchange among organ procurement organizations seems to be essential and has a direct positive impact on the chances of patients to get a timely, often life-saving transplantation [5]. All these efforts have, however, not resulted in a decreasing waiting time on the waiting list.

Fueled by the uncertainty and the time required to get a donor heart, mechanical circulatory support (MCS) as a bridge to transplantation (BTT) became mandatory to overcome death on the waiting list. Historically, MCS was developed if weaning from cardiopulmonary bypass (CPB) was not possible to allow for a recovery. Therefore, all centers performing congenital heart surgery have experience with extracorporeal membrane oxygenation (ECMO). Its use, however, is timely limited (days to weeks) before serious complications like bleeding occur [6]. Further, ECMO application is limited to short-term support due to immobilization of the patient and the patient must remain on the intensive care unit (ICU). Ventricular assist device (VAD) was shown to be superior to ECMO support, considering the increased risk of 1-year mortality associated with EMCO support [6, 7].

While VAD use in children is gaining more attention, there are several challenges to consider. On anatomical and physiological grounds, three different groups can be distinguished: adult patients with anatomic normal heart, pediatric patients with anatomic normal hearts, and patients with congenital heart disease (CHD) irrespective of age. There are clear differences in the pathophysiology of HF compared between adults, children, and CHD patients. Hospitalization of children suffering from HF due to CHD is increasing [1], while reported survival of children on VAD support suffering from CHD is still low [8, 9].

In adults with structural normal hearts, there is a large variety of different VADs which have proven to be safe for long-term support [10] and have developed as a standard treatment option [11]. For pediatrics, only a few VADs are available for patients with a body surface area (BSA) of less than 1.2 m^2 or weight less than 20 kg [12]. Furthermore, limited data are available as children are excluded in major VAD trials. Only one prospective trail is reported by Fraser et al. using the Berlin Heart EXCOR®. Currently, there are only two VADs designed for children with a body surface area below 1.2 m^2: the Medos HIS and the Berlin Heart EXCOR. Finally, in adult patients, the numbers of BiVAD implantations are declining [13, 14]; the incidence of biventricular failure among children remains high, with over 15% requiring BiVAD or total artificial heart support [15] and results seem to be inferior to LVAD only [16].

Finally, if a contraindication for HTx like pulmonary hypertension or malignancy is diagnosed, a concept known as bridge to transplantability may be considered.

All these considerations come with the need for care providers specialized in this field to determine optimal patient and device selection and to improve outcomes and decrease complication rates for new innovative strategies. This chapter focuses on durable VADs as BTT or candidacy in pediatrics.

2. Durable VAD support in children as BTT

In the 1970s, modifications of the original "heart-lung machine" like ECMO or extracorporeal centrifugal pumps [17] have been the principal art of cardiac support. With the need for real long-term support, the need for durable VADs became evident. In 1989, Frazier implanted a mechanical assist device in a 9-year-old boy who was successfully bridged to heart transplantation with a Biomedicus (Medtronic, Eden Prairie, MN) centrifugal pump; the supporting time was 12 h. In 1990, the first Berlin Heart EXCOR, in adult size 50-mL pump, was implanted in a 9-year-old child for 1 week with an uneventful postoperative time after heart transplantation [18]. Two years later, in 1992, pumps in sizes of 10, 25, and 30-mL have been devised, and the 10-mL pump was implanted in a 12-month-old child [19]. Two years later, the first Medos VAD (Medos Medizintechnik GmbH, Stolberg, Germany) was implanted successfully as bridge to transplantation [20]. In the last years, there has been an increase in the use of MCS in the pediatric population mainly driven by the development of smaller VADs, namely continuous flow (cf)-VADs.

2.1. Indication and device selection

Patient selection and timing remain crucial factors for improving outcomes in VAD recipients. In children with critical peripheral perfusion (i.e., metabolic acidosis; cardiac index of <2.0 l/ m^2/min, mixed venous oxygen saturation of <40%) despite inotropic support, early signs of renal, hepatic, or multiorgan failure without surgical options to correct any residual structural lesions should be considered for MCS. There are only a few contraindications for MCS like malignant neoplastic diseases with a very limited life expectancy, advanced multiorgan failure, complex congenital heart lesions involving intracardiac shunts or irreversible pulmonary failure and severe extracardiac malformations such as chromosomal and genetic syndromes with poor quality of life prognosis [21].

Selection differs significantly within the pediatric group by structural normal hearts or patients with CHD as well as the age and weight/size of the patient [15, 22, 23]. Some VADs are specified for its use in adults or pediatrics; some are licensed according to a specific body surface area (BsA) and/or some for specific weight/size. Contrarily to adults, where intracorporeal left ventricular assist device (LVAD) has become a routine treatment with subsequent discharge home, options for small children are still limited. A large variety of adult-sized ventricular assist devices (VADs) has proven to be safe for long-term support [10] but only a small number of VADs are available for patients with a body surface area (BSA) of less than 1.2 m^2 or weight less than 20 kg [12]. The Medos HIS (no longer on the market) and the Berlin Heart EXCOR are the only two devices currently designed for children with a body surface area below 1.2 m². The development of pediatric-specific cf-VADs (Infant Jarvik) is approved for Investigational Device Exemption by the US Food and Drug Administration on September 30, 2016 [24]. In adult-sized adolescents and some teenagers reaching a BsA of >1.2 m², the implantation of a continuous-flow (cf) intracorporeal device LVAD is feasible as results are non-inferior to extracorporeal devices [15, 25, 26] and discharge from hospital is possible which guaranties a better quality of life [15, 27–30].

2.2. Berlin Heart pediatric EXCOR

When speaking about pediatric VAD support, most data are available for Berlin Heart EXCOR (Berlin Heart AG, Berlin, Germany) (see **Figure 1**). It was specifically designed for small children and is a paracorporeal, pulsatile, pneumatically driven VAD usable

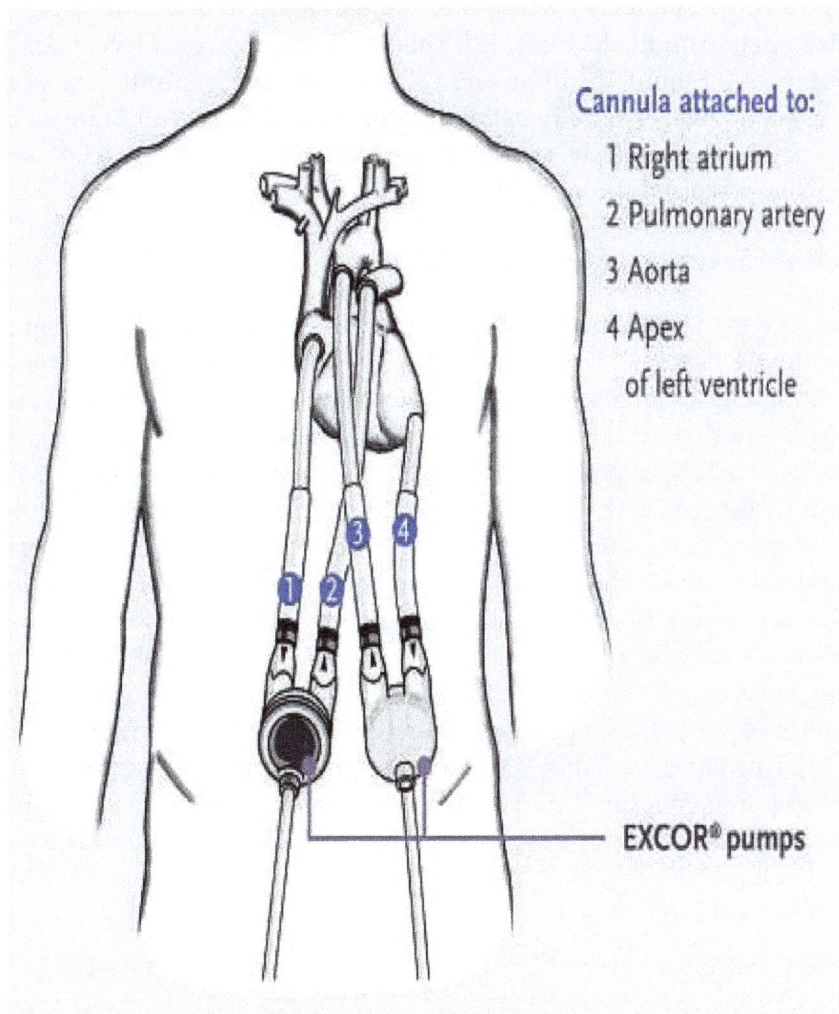

Cannula attached to:

1 Right atrium
2 Pulmonary artery
3 Aorta
4 Apex
  of left ventricle

EXCOR® pumps

Figure 1. The Berlin heart EXCOR (no permission was asked for reprint).

for left (LVAD) or biventricular (BiVAD) support. The EXCOR® ventricular assist device (EXCOR) is clinically used since 1990 for the circulatory support of pediatric heart failure in almost 2000 patients as BTT. The blood-contacting surfaces of EXCOR pumps are covalently coated with Heparin (CARMEDA CBAS®, Carmeda, Sweden) to enhance hemocompatibility. The system offers a spectrum of pumps with valves divided into a blood and air chamber and silicone cannula for every body size between 3 kg and adult size. The pump consists of a translucent, semi-rigid housing of polyurethane. The US investigational device exemption (IDE) multicenter trial examining the safety and efficacy of the device found a better survival for EXCOR compared to ECMO, and serious adverse events, including infection, stroke, and bleeding, were reported with 0.07 events per patient-day in the VAD group and with 0.08 events per patient-day in the ECMO group [6]. The EXCOR was first used in Europe, and the Berlin group gained great experience with the EXCOR even in neonates achieving a survival of 70% [31]. Nevertheless, the initial North American experience including 73 patients showed that younger age and BiVAD were significant risk factors for death while on the EXCOR [12]. This was confirmed by a recent study concluding that durable VADs should be used very cautiously in children suffering from complex CHD below 1 year of age, especially patients on previous ECMO and those who had prior cardiac surgery [23]. In this study, one-third of all EXCOR patients had CHD, and of these, 30% had a univentricular physiology [23].

2.3. Patients with congenital heart disease (CHD)

Patients, irrespective of age, with CHD represent a unique and difficult patient population to support with VAD/MCS. CHD represents a wide spectrum of cardiac anatomies including the special setting of single ventricle physiologies. Some of the children undergoing CHD surgery are not cured and remain at risk of developing end-stage heart failure. It is estimated that 10–20% of patients with CHD will require HTx at some point of their life. There is a variety of CHD that results in single ventricle physiology requiring surgical correction ending in the Fontan circulation. HF can occur at any time of the palliative surgery (Norwood stage I, bidirectional cavopulmonary anastomosis, Fontan completion). Large trials investigating the use of MCS in patients with single ventricle are missing. Mainly small series or case reports are published with high mortality rates (i.e., one of three patients surviving to discharge [32–34]) and adverse events, compared to a two-ventricular physiology [34]. Support for Glenn circulation has been proven with mixed results [33–36]. Currently available VADs are designed to provide support to the failing ventricle but requirements for VAD systems in the failing Fontan may require cavopulmonary. Nevertheless, available devices have been used for cavopulmonary support in failing Fontan patients [37–42]. For patients with failing Fontan circulation, TAH might be an option [43] (see subsequent text).

By contrast, VAD outcomes in adult CHD patients with two-ventricle physiology are comparable to non-ACHD patients. Most of these patients have a morphologic right ventricle working as systemic ventricle. VAD placement in these patients is possible, and some patients will benefit from VAD support [44–50].

2.4. Biventricular support (BiVAD, TAH)

The majority of implants in children are only for isolated left ventricular support. However, there is a certain percentage of patients (~17%) who require biventricular support with BiVAD or total artificial heart (TAH; see **Figure 2**) [15]. Results for BiVADS and for TAH (patients <21 years) have been reported to be inferior to LVAD only [16, 51]. The Berlin Heart EXCOR remains the "golden standard" for biventricular support in children due to size matters. Case reports and series using two cf-VADs in pediatrics (see **Figure 3**) with successful BTT with BSA as low as 0.6 m² have been published [52–55] even in patients with Fontan circulation [56].

2.5. Anticoagulation and monitoring

All patients on MCS/VAD support should receive anticoagulation (Class I recommendation) [11]. Thromboembolic events like stroke or pump thromboses in children supported with VAD remain serious adverse events and differ compared to adults [8, 57–59]. No standard anticoagulation protocol has been developed so far, and anticoagulation is tailored to different types of VAD and individualized by different centers. To achieve a balance between minimizing thromboembolic events and bleeding complications, an anticoagulation monitoring involving the international normalized ratio (INR), the thrombocyte aggregation test (TAT), and thromboelastography (TEG) has been proposed. The monitoring of unfractionated heparin remains a matter of discussion.

The initial North American EXCOR experience included no consistent anticoagulation protocol [6]. As for the US investigational device trial for the EXCOR, the investigators agreed on the Edmonton protocol. Briefly, this protocol uses a three-drug regimen involving aspirin,

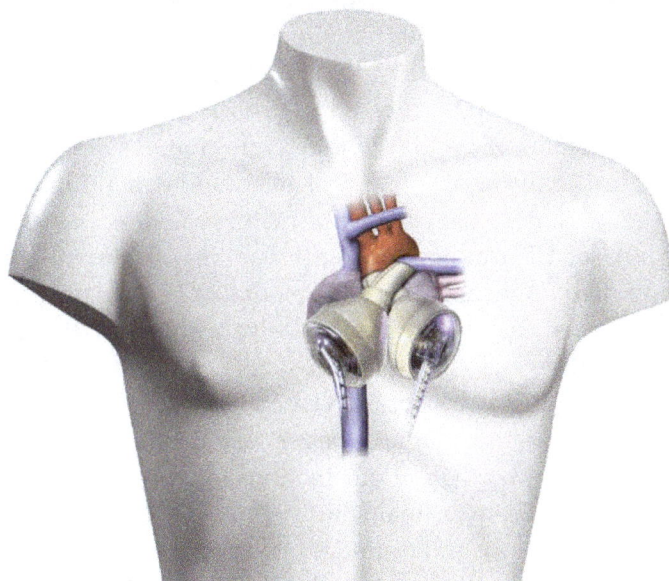

Figure 2. The Cardiowest is a total artificial heart provided by Snycardia (Tucson, AZ, USA). (http://www.syncardia.com/Medical-Professionals/compare-to-bivads.html) (no permission was asked for reprint).

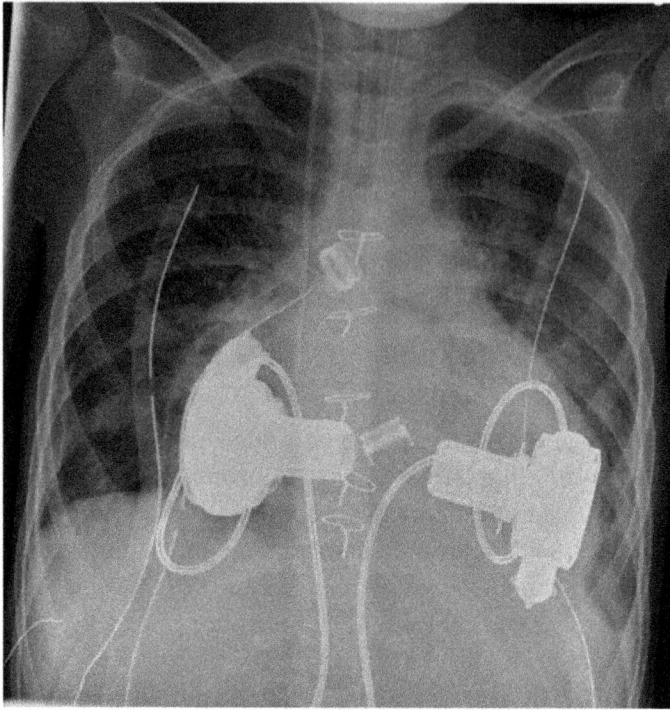

Figure 3. Two intracorporeal VADs for biventricular support in a child with a body weight of 27 kg (no permission was asked for reprint).

persantine, and enoxaparin or oral anticoagulation [12]. In the immediate postoperative period, unfractionated heparin (UFH) continues to be the anticoagulant of choice, especially in the early postoperative phase in which close titration is required [60]. While the use of UFH is unquestioned, monitoring remains a matter of discussion. Traditionally, in percutaneous coronary intervention or cardiac surgery, the effect of UFH is monitored by the aPTT or the ACT, when higher doses are used in conjunction with extracorporeal bypass. Although aPTT seems to be the standard criterion, it is known that aPTT is susceptible to physiological and nonphysiological factors and may under- or overestimate the level of anticoagulation. For this reason, plasma heparin assays—which determine the anticoagulation activity of UFH by measuring the ability of heparin-bound AT to inhibit FXa—have been proposed. Published data suggest that anti-Xa monitoring achieves therapeutic anticoagulation more rapidly, maintains the values within the goal range for a longer time, and requires fewer adjustments in dosage and repeated tests [61]; further, the aPTT is impacted more frequently by preanalytic compared to anti-Xa [62]. It also may be of particular advantage in pediatric patients (better correlated with heparin dosing than the aPTT or ACT in pediatric ECMO). We at our institution use anti-XA [63], but so far there are too less data available to draw a final solution and both methods are used clinically. After the removal of invasive lines and drainages, long-term anticoagulation with warfarin with a targeted INR and additional antiplatelet therapy can be started. Recently, a report has been published showing fewer strokes in pediatric EXCOR patients using a triple antiplatelet regimen [64].

While the proportion of patients who develop neurological dysfunction after implantation of pulsatile devices has been documented to be approximately 19–30%, the incidence of cerebral strokes in children supported by cf-VADs has not been well explored. A recent report from EUROMACS suggests that it may be as low as 0.1 events per patient year [29]. Similar to the EXCOR, UFH is started postoperatively and then switched to oral anticoagulation. Antiplatelet therapy is in most cases necessary and seems to be meaningful as the pump chamber lays intracorporeal.

3. Conclusions

Prolonged durable support in children of all ages and patients with CHD with VADs permits good survival to transplantation. While the Berlin Heart EXCOR remains the "golden standard" for small children, if biventricular is needed, and in some CHD scenarios, an increased miniaturization of VADs has increased cf-device use in these patient. Still, patient and device selection in these patients remain challenging and come with the need for care providers specialized in the field of pediatric/CHD MCS/VAD treatment.

Conflict of interest

The author does not have any conflict of interest concerning this chapter.

Appendices and nomenclature

BiVAD	biventricular assist device
CHD	congenital heart disease
ECMO	extracorporeal membrane oxygenation
EXCOR	Berlin Heart pediatric EXCOR
HF	heart failure
HTx	heart transplantation
LVAD	left ventricular assist device
MCS	mechanical circulatory support
UFH	unfractionated heparin
TAH	total artificial heart
VAD	ventricular assist device

Author details

Martin Schweiger and Michael Huebler

Address all correspondence to: martinl.schweigerr@kispi.uzh.ch

Department of Congenital Cardiovascular Surgery, University Children's Hospital, Zurich, Switzerland

References

[1] Adachi I, Fraser Jr CD. Mechanical circulatory support for infants and small children. Seminars in Thoracic and Cardiovascular Surgery. Pediatric Cardiac Surgery Annual. 2011;**14**(1):38-44

[2] Almond CS et al. Waiting list mortality among children listed for heart transplantation in the United States. Circulation. 2009;**119**(5):717-727

[3] West LJ et al. ABO-incompatible heart transplantation in infants. The New England Journal of Medicine. 2001;**344**(11):793-800

[4] Schweiger M et al. Pediatric heart transplantation. The Journal of Thoracic Disease. 2015;**7**(3):552-559

[5] Weiss J, Kocher M, Immer FF. International collaboration and organ exchange in Switzerland. The Journal of Thoracic Disease. 2015;**7**(3):543-548

[6] Fraser Jr CD et al. Prospective trial of a pediatric ventricular assist device. The New England Journal of Medicine. 2012;**367**(6):532-541

[7] Dipchand AI et al. The registry of the international society for heart and lung transplantation: Eighteenth official pediatric heart transplantation report—2015; focus theme: Early graft failure. The Journal of Heart and Lung Transplantation. 2015;**34**(10):1233-1243

[8] Reinhartz O et al. Multicenter experience with the thoratec ventricular assist device in children and adolescents. The Journal of Heart and Lung Transplantation. 2001;**20**(4):439-448

[9] Blume ED et al. Outcomes of children bridged to heart transplantation with ventricular assist devices: A multi-institutional study. Circulation. 2006;**113**(19):2313-2319

[10] Krabatsch T et al. Improvements in implantable mechanical circulatory support systems: Literature overview and update. Herz. 2011;**36**(7):622-629

[11] Feldman D et al. The 2013 international society for heart and lung transplantation guidelines for mechanical circulatory support: Executive summary. The Journal of Heart and Lung Transplantation. 2013;**32**(2):157-187

[12] Morales DL et al. Bridging children of all sizes to cardiac transplantation: The initial multicenter North American experience with the Berlin Heart EXCOR ventricular assist device. The Journal of Heart and Lung Transplantation. 2011;**30**(1):1-8

[13] Kirklin JK et al. The Fourth INTERMACS Annual Report: 4000 implants and counting. The Journal of Heart and Lung Transplantation. 2012;**31**(2):117-126

[14] Krabatsch T et al. Mechanical circulatory support-results, developments and trends. Journal of Cardiovascular Translational Research. 2011;**4**(3):332-339

[15] Blume ED et al. Second annual pediatric interagency registry for mechanical circulatory support (Pedimacs) report: Pre-implant characteristics and outcomes. Journal of Heart and Lung Transplantation. 2017;**37**(1):38-45

[16] Fan Y et al. Factors associated with the need of biventricular mechanical circulatory support in children with advanced heart failure. European Journal of Cardio-Thoracic Surgery. 2013;**43**(5):1028-1035

[17] Karl TR, Horton SB, Brizard C. Postoperative support with the centrifugal pump ventricular assist device (VAD). Seminars in Thoracic and Cardiovascular Surgery. Pediatric Cardiac Surgery Annual. 2006;**9**(1):83-91

[18] Warnecke H et al. Mechanical left ventricular support as a bridge to cardiac transplantation in childhood. European Journal of Cardio-Thoracic Surgery. 1991;**5**(6):330-333

[19] Hetzer R et al. Mechanical cardiac support in the young with the Berlin Heart EXCOR pulsatile ventricular assist device: 15 years' experience. Seminars in Thoracic and Cardiovascular Surgery. Pediatric Cardiac Surgery Annual. 2006;**9**:99-108

[20] Konertz W et al. Clinical experience with the MEDOS HIA-VAD system in infants and children: A preliminary report. The Annals of Thoracic Surgery. 1997;**63**(4):1138-1144

[21] Schweiger M et al. Paediatric ventricular assist devices: Current achievements. Swiss Medical Weekly. 2013;**143**:w13804

[22] Conway J et al. Delineating survival outcomes in children <10 kg bridged to transplant or recovery with the Berlin Heart EXCOR Ventricular Assist Device. JACC Heart Fail. 2015;**3**(1):70-77

[23] Morales DL et al. Berlin Heart EXCOR use in patients with congenital heart disease. The Journal of Heart and Lung Transplantation. 2017;**36**(11):1209-1216

[24] Adachi I et al. The miniaturized pediatric continuous-flow device: Preclinical assessment in the chronic sheep model. The Journal of Thoracic and Cardiovascular Surgery. 2017;**154**(1):291-300

[25] Cabrera AG et al. Outcomes of pediatric patients supported by the HeartMate II left ventricular assist device in the United States. The Journal of Heart and Lung Transplantation. 2013;**32**(11):1107-1113

[26] Conway J et al. Global experience with the Heartware HVAD® in pediatric patients: A preliminary analysis. JHLT. 2016;**35**(4S):1

[27] Conway J et al. Now how do we get them home? Outpatient care of pediatric patients on mechanical circulatory support. Pediatric Transplantation. 2016;**20**(2):194-202

[28] Schweiger M et al. Outpatient management of intra-corporeal left ventricular assist device system in children: A multi-center experience. American Journal of Transplantation. 2015;**15**(2):453-460

[29] Schweiger M et al. Cerebral strokes in children on intracorporeal ventricular assist devices: Analysis of the EUROMACS registry. European Journal of Cardio-Thoracic Surgery. 2018;**53**(2):416-421

[30] Blume ED et al. Outcomes of children implanted with ventricular assist devices in the United States: First analysis of the pediatric interagency registry for mechanical circulatory support (PediMACS). The Journal of Heart and Lung Transplantation. 2016;**35**(5):578-584

[31] Stiller B et al. Pneumatic pulsatile ventricular assist devices in children under 1 year of age. European Journal of Cardio-Thoracic Surgery. 2005;**28**(2):234-239

[32] Poh CL et al. Ventricular assist device support in patients with single ventricles: The Melbourne experience. Interactive Cardiovascular and Thoracic Surgery. 2017;**25**(2):310-316

[33] Adachi I et al. Outpatient management of a child with bidirectional Glenn shunts supported with implantable continuous-flow ventricular assist device. The Journal of Heart and Lung Transplantation. 2016;**35**(5):688-690

[34] Weinstein S et al. The use of the Berlin Heart EXCOR in patients with functional single ventricle. The Journal of Thoracic and Cardiovascular Surgery. 2014;**147**(2):697-704 (discussion 704-5)

[35] Irving CA et al. Successful bridge to transplant with the Berlin Heart after cavopulmonary shunt. The Journal of Heart and Lung Transplantation. 2009;**28**(4):399-401

[36] Adachi I et al. Mechanically assisted Fontan completion: A new approach for the failing Glenn circulation due to isolated ventricular dysfunction. The Journal of Heart and Lung Transplantation. 2016;**35**(11):1380-1381

[37] Throckmorton AL et al. A viable therapeutic option: Mechanical circulatory support of the failing Fontan physiology. Pediatric Cardiology. 2013;**34**(6):1357-1365

[38] Giridharan GA et al. Performance evaluation of a pediatric viscous impeller pump for Fontan cavopulmonary assist. The Journal of Thoracic and Cardiovascular Surgery. 2013; **145**(1):249-257

[39] Haggerty CM et al. Experimental and numeric investigation of Impella pumps as cavopulmonary assistance for a failing Fontan. The Journal of Thoracic and Cardiovascular Surgery. 2012;**144**(3):563-569

[40] Pretre R et al. Right-sided univentricular cardiac assistance in a failing Fontan circulation. The Annals of Thoracic Surgery. 2008;**86**(3):1018-1020

[41] Rodefeld MD et al. Cavopulmonary assist for the univentricular Fontan circulation: Von Karman viscous impeller pump. The Journal of Thoracic and Cardiovascular Surgery. 2010;**140**(3):529-536

[42] Pace Napoleone C et al. Ventricular assist device in a failing total cavopulmonary connection: A new step-by-step approach. Interactive Cardiovascular and Thoracic Surgery. 2017;**26**(2):341-342

[43] Wells D, Villa CR, Simon Morales DL. The 50/50 cc total artificial heart trial: Extending the benefits of the total artificial heart to underserved populations. Seminars in Thoracic and Cardiovascular Surgery. Pediatric Cardiac Surgery Annual. 2017;**20**:16-19

[44] Steiner JM et al. Durable mechanical circulatory support in teenagers and adults with congenital heart disease: A systematic review. International Journal of Cardiology. 2017; **245**:135-140

[45] Stokes MB et al. Successful bridge to Orthotopic cardiac transplantation with implantation of a HeartWare HVAD in management of systemic right ventricular failure in a patient with transposition of the great arteries and previous atrial switch procedure. Heart, Lung & Circulation. 2016;**25**(5):e69-e71

[46] VanderPluym CJ et al. Outcomes following implantation of mechanical circulatory support in adults with congenital heart disease: An analysis of the interagency registry for mechanically assisted circulatory support (INTERMACS). Journal of Heart and Lung Transplantation. 2017;**37**(1):89-99

[47] Tanoue Y, Jinzai Y, Tominaga R. Jarvik 2000 axial-flow ventricular assist device placement to a systemic morphologic right ventricle in congenitally corrected transposition of the great arteries. Journal of Artificial Organs. 2016;**19**(1):97-99

[48] Maly J et al. Bridge to transplantation with long-term mechanical assist device in adults after the mustard procedure. The Journal of Heart and Lung Transplantation. 2015;**34**(9):1177-1181

[49] Dakkak AR et al. Implanting a nonpulsatile axial flow left ventricular assist device as a bridge to transplant for systemic ventricular failure after a mustard procedure. Experimental and Clinical Transplantation. 2015;**13**(5):485-487

[50] Schweiger M et al. Biventricular failure in dextro-transposition of the great arteries corrected with the Mustard procedure: VAD support of the systemic ventricle is enough. The International Journal of Artificial Organs. 2015;**38**:233-235

[51] Morales DLS et al. Worldwide experience with the Syncardia Total artificial heart in the pediatric population. ASAIO Journal. 2017;**63**(4):518-519

[52] Glass L et al. Continuous-flow, implantable biventricular assist device as bridge to cardiac transplantation in a small child with restrictive cardiomyopathy. Journal of Heart and Lung Transplantation. 2017;**37**(1):173-174

[53] Stein ML et al. HeartWare HVAD for biventricular support in children and adolescents: The Stanford experience. ASAIO Journal. 2016;**62**(5):e46-e51

[54] Schweiger M et al. Biventricular intracorporeal ventricular assist device in a 10-year-old child. The International Journal of Artificial Organs. 2016;**39**(1):48-50

[55] Peng E et al. An extended role of continuous flow device in pediatric mechanical circulatory support. The Annals of Thoracic Surgery. 2016;**102**(2):620-627

[56] Ovroutski S et al. Two pumps for single ventricle: Mechanical support for establishment of biventricular circulation. The Annals of Thoracic Surgery. 2017;**104**(2):e143-e145

[57] Fan Y et al. Outcomes of ventricular assist device support in young patients with small body surface area. European Journal of Cardio-Thoracic Surgery. 2011;**39**(5):699-704

[58] Reinhartz O et al. Thoratec ventricular assist devices in pediatric patients: Update on clinical results. ASAIO Journal. 2005;**51**(5):501-503

[59] Schweiger M et al. Complication profile of the Berlin Heart EXCOR biventricular support in children. Artificial Organs. 2013;**37**:730-735

[60] Schechter T et al. Unfractionated heparin dosing in young infants: Clinical outcomes in a cohort monitored with anti-factor Xa levels. Journal of Thrombosis and Haemostasis. 2012;**10**(3):368-374

[61] Guervil DJ et al. Activated partial thromboplastin time versus antifactor Xa heparin assay in monitoring unfractionated heparin by continuous intravenous infusion. The Annals of Pharmacotherapy. 2011;**45**(7-8):861-868

[62] Schweiger M, Hubler M, Albisetti M. Heparin anticoagulation monitoring in patients supported by ventricular assist devices. ASAIO Journal. 2015;**61**(5):487-488

[63] Schweiger M et al. Acute chemotherapy-induced cardiomyopathy treated with intracorporeal left ventricular assist device in an 8-year-old child. ASAIO Journal. 2013;**59**(5): 520-522

[64] Rosenthal DN et al. Impact of a modified anti-thrombotic guideline on stroke in children supported with a pediatric ventricular assist device. The Journal of Heart and Lung Transplantation. 2017;**36**(11):1250-1257

3

Post-Heart Transplantation Lymphoproliferations

Sylvain Choquet

Abstract

Post-transplant lymphoproliferations (PTLDs) are the cancer with the highest incidence after cardiac transplantation. The World Health Organization (WHO) has defined several specific entities: clonal or non-clonal, early, polymorphic or monomorphic. Early PTLDs being generally positive for Epstein-Barr virus (EBV), preventive and preemptive treatments have been proposed; the former did not lead to effective attitudes, unlike preemptive treatment, based on EBV viral load monitoring the first year, which proposes a decrease of the immunosuppression with or without rituximab according to the viral load and the answer to the immunosuppression decrease. The curative treatment of CD20 positive PTLDs, the most frequent form, begins to be codified; it starts with a decrease in immunosuppression and then uses rituximab monotherapy and, depending on the response, either only rituximab or four courses of R-CHOP. By following this management, the incidence of early PTLDs decreases and the treatment of PTLDs provides survivals close to that of other transplant patients.

Keywords: post-transplant lymphoproliferation, epstein barr virus, lymphoma, rituximab

1. Introduction

Non-Hodgkin's lymphoma (NHL) is the cancer with the highest incidence after cardiac transplantation. However, NHL is only part of the PTLD, the WHO recognizing several entities, whose lymphomatous and/or clonal appearance is not systematic. Since PTLDs are often linked to Epstein-Barr virus (EBV), preventive and above all preemptive treatments have been proposed to reduce the incidence of these proliferations. The prognosis of PTLD is generally presented as severe; however, the latest therapeutic proposals, adapted to the response to rituximab, provide survivals close to those of the rest of the population of transplanted patients.

2. Epidemiology

It is usual in the literature to estimate between 3 and 5% the risk of a cardiac-transplanted patient developing a PTLD [1]; however, these figures are old and vary depending on immunosuppression and duration of patients' lives, fortunately improved in the last 10 years. The largest study on the epidemiology of PTLD [2] involved 175,732 organ transplants between 1987 and 2008, including 10% of heart transplants. Pulmonary cancers represent the most frequent cancers (386/100,000/years) just in front of the NHL (283/100,000/years) but the standardized incidence ratio (SIR) of the NHL is very clearly superior to that of all the other cancers. **Table 1** presents the incidence and the SIR of the main cancers according to the transplanted organ. The risk of PTLD persists as long as immunosuppression is used, that is, until death for cardiac transplant patients; it is maximum the first year after transplantation, with an SIR greater than 10, but remains stable thereafter, with a SIR between 3 and 10 for a follow-up of up to 15 years.

Transplanted organ	Cancer: incidence (100,000/years)/SIR			
	NHL	Lung cancer	Liver cancer	Kidney cancer
Heart	283/7.79	386/2.67	13.8/1.02	90.1/2.90
Kidney	141/6.05	115/1.46	10.7/1.08	126/6.66
Liver	217/7.77	178/1.95	495/44	39.9/1.80
Lung	532/18.73	626/6.13	17/2.04	34/1.49

Table 1. Incidence and SIR of the main cancers developed after transplantation depending on the transplanted organ.

EBV, initially described as always associated with PTLDs, is actually only half of the time. Almost always found in children, most often on the occasion of a primary infection, and in early forms (before the first year after transplantation), it has become rare in the late forms, the most common situation of our days [3]. In cerebral PTLDs, representing 10% of PTLDs, EBV is almost always found [4].

3. Diagnosis

3.1. Definition: anatomopathology

PTLDs, as their name suggests, are lymphoid proliferations occurring after solid or hematopoietic organ transplantation and are authentic entities recognized in the WHO classification [5], presented in **Table 2**. We will retain some peculiarities to this classification:

- Early lesions are almost always EBV positive.

- Polymorphic lesions (infiltration by cells of different types) are polyclonal in almost half of the cases.

- Monomorphic lesions are clonal.

- The cerebral PTLDs are almost always monomorphic B lesions.

- B-type diffuse B-cell monomorphic lesions are by far the most common PTLD.

- Follicular lymphomas, marginal zone lymphomas, and mantle cell lymphomas are not considered PTLDs even when they occur after transplantation.

Early lesions	Plasmacytic hyperplasia PTLD
	Infectious mononucleosis PTLD
Florid follicular hyperplasia PTLD	
Polymorphic PTLD	
Monomorphic B PTLD	Diffuse large B cell lymphoma
	Burkitt lymphoma
	Plasmacytoma-like
Monomorphic T PTLD	T-cell lymphoma, non-otherwise specified
	Hepatosplenic T-cell lymphoma
	T/NK lymphoma
Classical Hodgkin lymphoma PTLD	

Table 2. WHO classification for PTLD.

3.2. Diagnosis and extension assessment

The presentation of PTLDs is not unambiguous and the signs are not specific. In early forms, an alteration of the general status with fever is often present. In the other forms, the clinical signs depend on the tumoral localizations; for this reason, the digestive localizations are frequent and can be a source of digestive disorders, pain, even perforation, or necrosis (**Figure 1**).

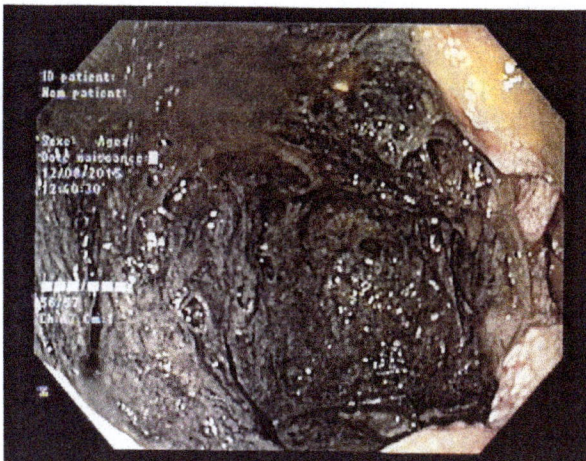

Figure 1. Gut necrosis due to a PTLD.

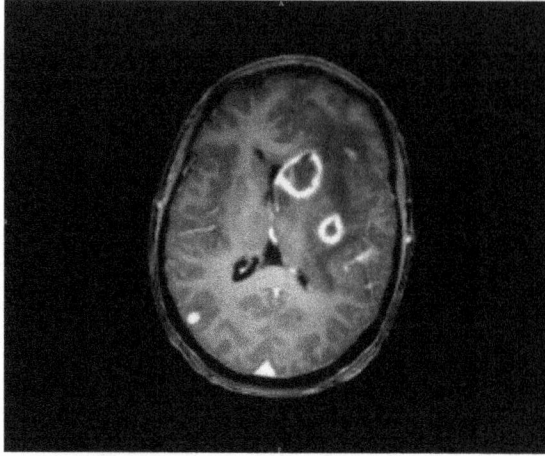

Figure 2. Cerebral PTLD, MRI in T1 with gadolinium.

Paraclinically, the EBV viral load (EVL) is essential, and a high rate is in favor of an EBV-positive PTLD; it is also a good marker of response during treatment. Imaging, CT scanning, or especially PET-CT scan are diagnostic [6] and allow an adequate extension assessment. The appearance of tumors and nodes is similar to that of lymphomas of immunocompetent patients. In the particular case of cerebral PTLD, the lesions are necrotic, in the form of a cockade, identical to toxoplasmic lesions, as in patients with HIV (**Figure 2**). MRI spectrometry can point to PTLD rather than infection. In the absence of contraindication, a lumbar puncture is necessary; it must include a cytology with anti-CD20 labeling on a slide, a phenotyping, a search for B clonality, and an EBV viral load. If lumbar puncture is found in lymphoma cells, cerebral biopsy is not necessary.

4. Treatment

4.1. Preventive treatment

Preventive treatment is defined as a systematic treatment that can avoid or reduce the incidence of PTLDs; it only concerns EBV-positive PTLDs. In this area, no study specifically targets heart-transplant patients. The interest of antivirals, especially ganciclovir, does not seem to be confirmed. On the other hand, polyvalent CMV immunoglobulins (in fact rich in anti-EBV immunoglobulins) have shown, in a retrospective study, an interest in kidney-transplant patients, suppressing the risk of PTLD occurring during the year of prevention in more than 2000 patients [7], whereas no preventive effect was detected in patients receiving ganciclovir. However, a prospective study, admittedly of a smaller size, did not show any difference between a preventive treatment with ganciclovir + placebo versus ganciclovir + immunoglobulins against CMV [8]. Currently, no preventive treatment is recommended in cardiac-transplant patients.

4.2. Preemptive treatment

Preemptive treatment only concerns EBV-positive PTLDs; it consists of treating patients according to their EBV viral load. It is based on the fact that the majority of EBV-positive

PTLDs are preceded by an increase in EBV load or a simple positivity in the case of primary infections [8]. The most classic attitude is to reduce immunosuppression, where possible [9–11]. As the EBV reservoir is the B lymphocyte, rituximab has also been used successfully in this setting, especially after allografts of hematopoietic stem cells [12]. Much less available and usable only in the context of protocols, anti EBV T lymphocytes, either autologous (taken from the patient and stimulated ex vivo) [13, 14], or allogeneic (from healthy donor lymphocyte banks) [15], have been used effectively in case of EBV reactivation. Specifically developed in cardiac-transplant patients, a treatment algorithm has been validated on nearly 300 patients whose immunosuppression was identical [16]; it is based initially on the serological status before transplant and then on the EVL carried out at each follow-up visit, for at least 1 year. The algorithm is described in **Figure 3**. In summary, immunosuppression is reduced as soon as the EVL is positive if the recipient was seronegative, since it is then a primary EBV infection, that is, when the EVL is greater than 10^5 copies/ml in other case.

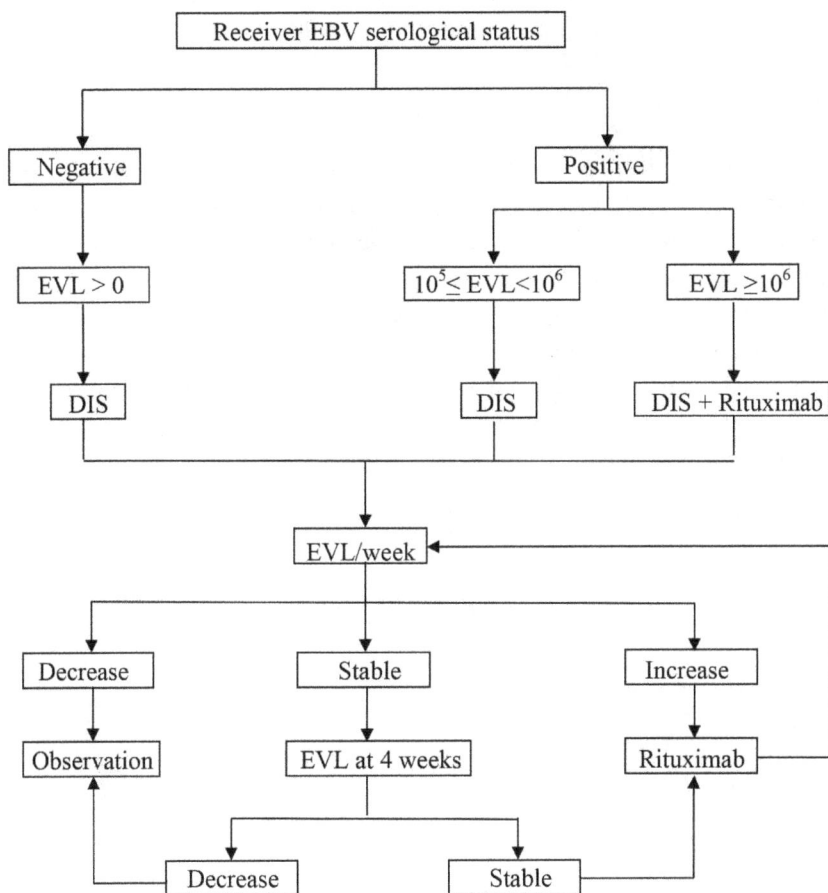

EVL = EBV viral load (copies/ml)
DIS = decrease of immunosuppression
Rituximab = one injection of 375 mg/m² IV

Figure 3. Algorithm for preemptive treatment of PTLD after heart transplantation, depending on serological status and EBV viral load.

An injection of 375 mg/m^2 of rituximab is performed, in addition to the decrease in immunosuppression, if the EVL is greater than 10^6 copies/ml, or if the initial decrease in immunosuppression fails. No cases of EBV-positive PTLD were diagnosed in this series, which is statistically significant in historical comparison with more than 800 patients transplanted in the same unit before using this algorithm.

4.3. PTLD treatment

4.3.1. Decrease of the immunosuppression

The decrease in immunosuppression remains the benchmark for the initial management of PTLDs. It allows complete response in less than 10% of cases, mainly in early forms [17, 18]. As the median time of response is 3.6 months [19], it is conventional to wait 4 weeks before evaluating the response to the decrease of immunosuppression, except in case of progression. Even in the event of failure, it is necessary to keep the immunosuppression as low as possible because it seems to potentiate immunochemotherapy [20].

4.3.2. Immunochemotherapy

In the case of failure of the reduction of immunosuppression, in CD20-positive PTLDs, which represents the vast majority of cases, sequential immunochemotherapy is the reference treatment, validated by two European prospective studies [3, 21]. The processing algorithm is shown in **Figure 4**. The first phase is to use only rituximab monotherapy and wait 3 weeks before evaluating the response, in case of complete remission, which is found in one-third of cases; rituximab is continued alone, this to avoid chemotherapy, in other cases, R-CHOP (rituximab, cyclophosphamide, doxorubicin, vincristine, prednisone) is used, a reference chemotherapy of NHL, but only for four cures against six to eight in the immunocompetent patients, and a case is presented in **Figure 5**. This therapeutic attitude gives 88% of response, 70% of complete response, and a median survival of 6.6 years, which currently constitutes the best results of the literature for a prospective study. In pediatric patients, lightened chemotherapy regimens have been proposed, without doxorubicin or vincristine, making it possible to obtain an overall survival of 83% at 2 years and an event-free survival of 71% [22].

4.4. Specific PTLDs

4.4.1. PTLD of the central nervous system

PTLDs in the central nervous system account for 10% of PTLDs, and even if they occur mostly after kidney transplants, they are not uncommon after cardiac transplantation. Their management is not consensual but should include if possible a reduction of immunosuppression and methotrexate adapted to the renal function, and the addition of aracytine and rituximab is recommended. In case of failure or contraindication, radiotherapy is an option. In a recent retrospective study, the response rate was 60% but the 3-year survival was only 43% [4].

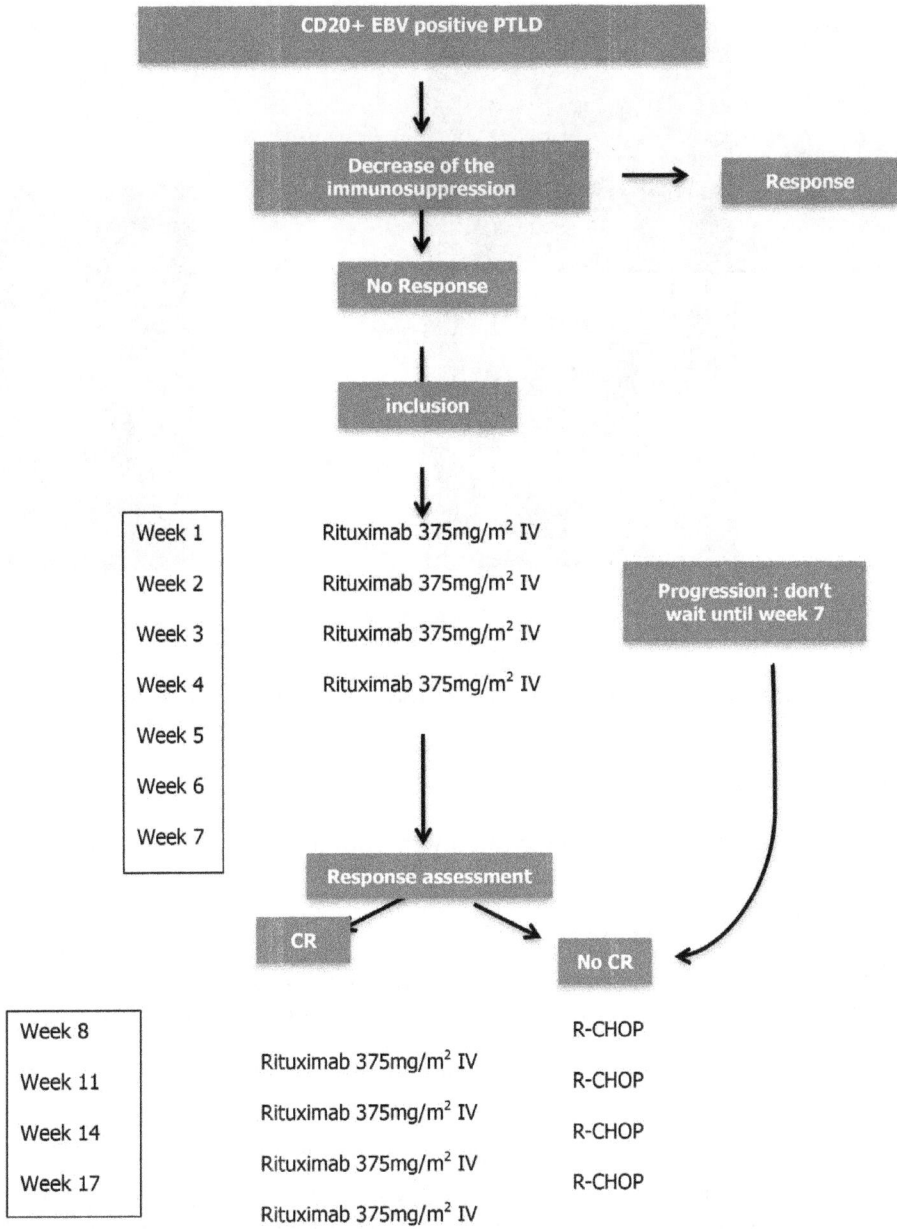

Figure 4. Algorithm to treat CD20-positive PTLD in first line.

4.4.2. Classical Hodgkin PTLD

Hodgkin PTLD should be treated as Hodgkin's immunocompetent patients, without rituximab (Hodgkin's are CD20 negative); their prognosis is excellent.

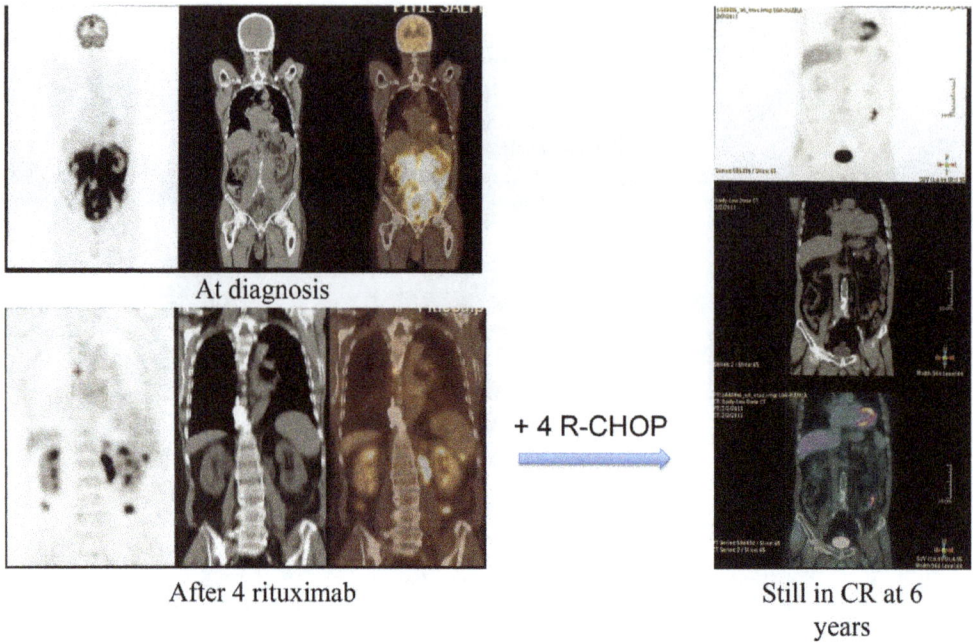

Figure 5. Response of a monomorphic diffuse large B cell PTLD after four rituximab and after four R-CHOP.

4.4.3. Plasmacytic hyperplasia PTLD

This rare form of early lesions can be treated with radiotherapy or lymphoma chemotherapy.

4.4.4. T-cell lymphoma PTLD

This type of PTLD has a very poor prognosis, rituximab is useless and the classic chemotherapy-type CHOP has little effectiveness. In case of localized form, radiotherapy may be useful.

4.4.5. Relapses

Relapses after complete remission are rare; if they occur late after the first PTLD, a comparison of the clones is necessary because a second PTLD, independent of the first one, is possible; if it is the case, the algorithm of first line, describes previously, can be reused, and the maximum dose of anthracycline will not be reached. In other cases, NHL treatments of immunocompetent patients in relapse may be used, even hematopoietic stem cell autograft.

4.5. Cell therapy

Cell therapy is not yet available outside study protocols. Its principle is to use T cells specifically directed against EBV antigens, so it is only applicable to half of PTLDs. It is mostly the allogeneic lymphocyte banks, from healthy donors, that are promising. The lymphocytes are selected according to the HLA typing of the tumor. In the Scottish experience, 12 complete remissions were obtained from 33 treated patients, but many of these patients had not received rituximab in the first line [23]. The ATARA Biotherapeutics laboratory begins in 2018, a phase 3 study using allogeneic anti-EBV lymphocytes against placebo in relapsed or refractory PTLDs, which could allow in the medium term to offer this therapy to all centers treating PTLDs.

4.6. CAR-T cells and anti-PD1/anti-PDL1

CAR-T cells, which are being developed in lymphoid hemopathies of immunocompetent patients, have not yet been used in an immunocompromised context that could potentially reduce their effectiveness.

Anti-PD1/PDL1 antibodies by improving immunity expose patients to rejection of the transplanted organ, sometimes abruptly; their indication in PTLDs, mainly of Hodgkin type, is strongly discouraged and should only be proposed by the last resort [24].

5. Conclusion

PTLDs are a clearly defined entity, representing the most increased cancer among cardiac-transplant recipients compared to the general population. Its management, from preemptive treatment to curative treatment, has been considerably improved in order to obtain a survival rate similar to that of other transplant recipients. The treatment deviates significantly from that of immunocompetent lymphomas and requires management by teams accustomed to this type of pathology, both for the follow-up of the transplant and for the hematological treatment. The development of cell therapies is very likely the next step in progress.

Author details

Sylvain Choquet

Address all correspondence to: sylvain.choquet@aphp.fr

Service d'Hématologie Clinique, Hôpital de la Pitié-Salpêtrière, Paris, France

References

[1] Opelz G, Döhler B. Lymphomas after solid organ transplantation: A collaborative transplant study report. American Journal of Transplantation. 2004;4(2):222-230

[2] Engels EA, Pfeiffer RM, Fraumeni JF Jr, et al. Spectrum of cancer risk among US solid organ transplant recipients. Journal of the American Medical Association. 2011;306(17):1891-1901

[3] Trappe RU, Dierickx D, Zimmermann H, et al. Response to rituximab induction is a predictive marker in B-cell post-transplant lymphoproliferative disorder and allows successful stratification into rituximab or R-CHOP consolidation in an international, prospective, multicenter phase II trial. Journal of Clinical Oncology. 2017;35(5):536-543

[4] Evens AM, Choquet S, Kroll-Desrosiers AR, et al. Primary CNS post-transplant lymphoproliferative disease (PTLD): An international report of 84 cases in the modern era. American Journal of Transplantation. 2013;13(6):1512-1522

[5] Swerdlow SH, Campo E, Pileri SA, Harris NL, et al. The 2016 revision of the World Health Organization classification of lymphoid neoplasms. Blood. 2016;127(20):2375-2390

[6] Bianchi E, Pascual M, Nicod M, et al. Clinical usefulness of FDG-PET/CT scan imaging in the management of posttransplant lymphoproliferative disease. Transplantation. 2008;85(5):707-712

[7] Opelz G, Daniel V, Naujokat C, et al. Effect of cytomegalovirus prophylaxis with immunoglobulin or with antiviral drugs on post-transplant non-Hodgkin lymphoma: A multicentre retrospective analysis. The Lancet Oncology. 2007;8(3):212-218

[8] Humar A, Hebert D, Davies HD, et al. A randomized trial of ganciclovir versus ganciclovir plus immune globulin for prophylaxis against Epstein-Barr virus related posttransplant lymphoproliferative disorder. Transplantation. 2006;81(6):856-861

[9] Stevens SJ, Verschuuren EA, Pronk I, et al. Frequent monitoring of Epstein-Barr virus DNA load in unfractionated whole blood is essential for early detection of posttransplant lymphoproliferative disease in high-risk patients. Blood. 2001;97:1165-1171

[10] McDiarmid SV, Jordan S, Kim GS, et al. Prevention and preemptive therapy of postransplant lymphoproliferative disease in pediatric liver recipients. Transplantation. 1998;66:1604-1611

[11] Lee TC, Savoldo B, Rooney CM, et al. Quantitative EBV viral loads and immunosuppression alterations can decrease PTLD incidence in pediatric liver transplant recipients. American Journal of Transplantation. 2005;5(9):2222-2228

[12] Bakker NA, Verschuuren EA, Erasmus ME, et al. Epstein-Barr virus-DNA load monitoring late after lung transplantation: A surrogate marker of the degree of immunosuppression and a safe guide to reduce immunosuppression. Transplantation. 2007;83:433-438

[13] van Esser JW, Niesters HG, van der Holt B, et al. Prevention of Epstein-Barr virus-lymphoproliferative disease by molecular monitoring and preemptive rituximab in high-risk patients after allogeneic stem cell transplantation. Blood. 2002;99:4364-4369

[14] Comoli P, Labirio M, Basso S, et al. Infusion of autologous Epstein-Barr virus (EBV)-specific cytotoxic T cells for prevention of EBV-related lymphoproliferative disorder in solid organ transplant recipients with evidence of active virus replication. Blood. 2002;99:2592-2598

[15] Savoldo B, Goss JA, Hammer MM, et al. Treatment of solid organ transplant recipients with autologous Epstein Barr virus-specific cytotoxic T lymphocytes (CTLs). Blood. 2006;108:2942-2949

[16] Khanna R, Bell S, Sherritt M, Galbraith A, et al. Activation and adoptive transfer of Epstein-Barr virus-specific cytotoxic T cells in solid organ transplant patients with posttransplant lymphoproliferative disease. Proceedings of the National Academy of Sciences of the United States of America. 1999;**96**:10391-10396

[17] Choquet S, Varnous S, Deback C, et al. Adapted treatment of Epstein–Barr virus infection to prevent post-transplant lymphoproliferative disorder after heart transplantation. American Journal of Transplantation. 2014;**14**:857-866

[18] Starzl TE, Nalesnik MA, Porter KA, et al. Reversibility of lymphomas and lymphoproliferative lesions developing under cyclosporin-steroid therapy. Lancet. 1984;**1**(8377):583-587

[19] Schaar CG, van der Pijl JW, van Hoek B, et al. Successful outcome with a "quintuple approach" of posttransplant lymphoproliferative disorder. Transplantation. 2001;**71**: 47-52

[20] Tsai DE, Hardy CL, Tomaszewski JE, et al. Reduction in immunosuppression as initial therapy for posttransplant lymphoproliferative disorder: Analysis of prognostic variables and long-term follow-up of 42 adult patients. Transplantation. 2001;**71**:1076-1088

[21] Aull MJ, Buell JF, Trofe J, et al. Experience with 274 cardiac transplant recipients with posttransplant lymphoproliferative disorder: A report from the Israel Penn International Transplant Tumor Registry. Transplantation. 2004;**78**(11):1676-1682

[22] Trappe R, Oertel S, Leblond V, et al. Sequential treatment with rituximab followed by CHOP chemotherapy in adult B-cell post-transplant lymphoproliferative disorder (PTLD): The prospective international multicentre phase 2 PTLD-1 trial. The Lancet Oncology. 2012;**13**:196-206

[23] Gross TG, Orjuela MA, Perkins SL, et al. Low-dose chemotherapy and rituximab for posttransplant lymphoproliferative disease (PTLD): A Children's Oncology Group Report. American Journal of Transplantation. 2012;**12**:3069-3075

[24] Haque T, Wilkie GM, Jones MM, et al. Allogeneic cytotoxic T-cell therapy for EBV-positive posttransplantation lymphoproliferative disease: Results of a phase 2 multicenter clinical trial. Blood. 2007;**110**(4):1123-1131

[25] Kittai AS, Oldham H, Taylor M. Immune checkpoint inhibitors in organ transplant patients. Journal of Immunotherapy. 2017;**40**(7):277-281

4

Heart Transplant: Current Indications and Patient Selection

Ulises López-Cardoza, Carles Díez-López and
José González-Costello

Abstract

Heart transplant remains the gold standard treatment for end-stage heart failure, in spite of the recent advances in pharmacological treatment and device therapy. As expected, since the first heart transplant was performed 50 years ago, outcomes in heart transplant have continued to improve over the last decades focusing on perioperative management, the availability of newer and better mechanical circulatory support before and after heart transplant and immunosuppressive drug development. Nonetheless, in the last years we have witnessed a significant drop in the heart donor's pool as the greatest limiting factor, coupled with a rising number of advanced heart failure patients. Moreover, the difficulty in handling these patients, with multiple and more complex comorbidities, is continuously increasing. More importantly and despite these difficulties, conditional half-life in transplanted patients has nowadays reached 12 years of life expectancy. Thus, besides trying to increase donor numbers, candidate selection emerges as one of the most challenging issues for heart transplant programs. In this chapter we review the latest knowledge on indications for heart transplant, as well as the available screening and optimization tools in candidate selection in order to continue improving outcomes.

Keywords: heart transplant, indications, advanced heart failure, ventricular assist device

1. Introduction

Heart transplant (HTx) is indicated in patients with stage D heart failure (HF) who remain with severely disabling symptoms in spite of optimal medical and device treatment, and where other surgical options have been excluded [1]. In patients with progressive HF, treatment optimization by selection and up-titration of appropriate drugs (e.g., beta-blockers and inhibitors of the renin-angiotensin-aldosterone axis), device implantation (resynchronization therapy, implanted cardioverter defibrillator), and surgical intervention if appropriate (e.g., valve replacement in case of valve disease) becomes mandatory. Only in cases where conventional HF treatment is not well tolerated and/or the patient presents an unfavorable course we will raise the option of HTx. At this point, it is useful to recognize the clinical and hemodynamic parameters that identify patients in an advanced-HF (AHF) situation (**Table 1**), which represents 5% of the total number of patients in HF [2]. In the case of patients in cardiogenic shock (CS), the priority is to get the patient out of the shock situation and correct multi-organ failure, for which we will usually need inotropic and vasoactive treatment, intra-aortic balloon counterpulsation and, in some cases, ventricular mechanical assistance devices (VAD). Once the patient is stable, we will have to attempt to wean the VAD, if we consider that myocardial recovery is an option, or HTx otherwise.

The long waiting times and the increasing number of unstable patients have favored the development of mechanical circulatory support (MCS) therapies as bridge to transplant (BTT) and bridge to candidacy or decision (BTC/BTD). This was initially achieved by the use of short-term ventricular assist devices (STVADs), but in the last decades long-term ventricular assist

---

1. Severe symptoms of heart failure with dyspnea and/or fatigue at rest or on minimal exertion (NYHA functional class III or IV)

2. Episodes of fluid retention (pulmonary and/or systemic congestion, peripheral edema) and/or of reduced cardiac output at rest (peripheral hypoperfusion)

3. Objective evidence of severe cardiac dysfunction, shown by at least 1 of the following

   a. Low left ventricular ejection fraction (<30%)

   b. Pseudonormal or restrictive mitral inflow pattern on Doppler echocardiography

   c. High left ventricular filling pressures (mean PCWP >16 mmHg, and/or mean RAP >12 mmHg by pulmonary artery catheterization)

   d. High natriuretic peptide levels, in the absence of non-cardiac causes

4. Severe impairment of functional capacity shown by 1 of the following:

   a. Inability to exercise

   b. 6-minute walk test ≤300 m or less in females and/or patients aged ≥75 years

   c. Peak oxygen consumption <12 to 14 mL/kg/min

5. History of ≥1 heart failure hospitalization in the past 6 months

6. Presence of all the previous features despite "attempts to optimize" therapy including diuretics, renin-angiotensin-aldosterone system inhibitors, and beta-blockers, unless these are poorly tolerated or contraindicated, and cardiac resynchronization when indicated

---

NYHA: New York Heart Association; PCWP: pulmonary capillary wedge pressure; RAP: right atrial pressure.

Table 1. Definition of advanced heart failure according to ESC (Adapted from Metra et al. [2]).

devices (LTVADs) have been developed and allow for longer periods of support. Because recovery of the ventricular dysfunction is possible, especially in some settings such as myocarditis or acute coronary syndrome, the bridge to recovery (BTR) strategy is another option. Finally, the development of more reliable LTVADs has created the possibility of destination therapy (DT) in patients who are not candidates for HTx because of significant comorbidities. In this chapter we will focus our attention in the use of LTVADs as a bridge to transplant.

When evaluating a patient for HTx, we must assess the following aspects:

1. What is the expected mortality of the HF patient with the maximal surgical and medical treatment options?

2. What is the risk of performing a HTx? Which are the potential complications derived from the medical and immunosuppressive treatment after the intervention?

3. Who is the appropriate candidate? When should we put the patient on the waiting list for HTx?

4. How can we optimize our patient before HTx in order to improve post-operative outcomes?

2. Assessing prognosis of the patient with HF

In spite of the recent treatment advances, HF mortality is expected to be around 10% per year in large randomized studies [3], with a median survival of approximately 2 years in unselected cohorts [4]. Because mortality during the first year post-HTx ranges between 12 and 20% and the median of survival of the heart transplant is 12 years [5], it is important to carry out an adequate prognostic stratification in order to select those patients who will obtain the maximum benefit from HTx. Along these lines, we will review the most important clinical features and risk factors that should direct clinicians to undergo an early and comprehensive evaluation, and confirm if the patient is an appropriate candidate for the available advanced therapies, before a more severe deterioration is present and treatment options become compromised.

2.1. Clinical parameters

Multiple clinical parameters are associated with higher mortality in HF patients. During the last years, there has been a considerable effort by clinicians to define the common characteristics of AHF, and these can be seen in **Table 1**. For instance, progressive treatment intolerance, persistent clinical signs of HF, echocardiographic and hemodynamic signs of low output, multi-organ involvement and repeated hospitalizations, severely compromise patients' prognosis [6].

2.2. Etiology of heart failure

Ischemic cardiomyopathy has traditionally been associated with higher mortality, especially when severe left ventricular dysfunction and three-vessel or main stem left coronary artery disease unsuitable for revascularization is present [7]. Congenital heart diseases are also associated with greater mortality because of the higher degree of pulmonary arterial hypertension and possible previous cardiac surgeries [5]. Therefore, we recommend referring these patients to specific transplant centers with congenital heart disease expertise.

Cardiomyopathies are disorders in which the heart muscle is structurally and functionally abnormal in the absence of other causes such as coronary artery disease, arterial hypertension, valvular heart disease, congenital heart disease or any other condition that may cause abnormal loading conditions. In idiopathic dilated cardiomyopathies, the presence of a higher degree of fibrosis demonstrated by delayed gadolinium enhancement in cardiac magnetic resonance (MRI) is associated with worse prognosis and sudden death [8]. T1 and T2 mapping are MRI-based techniques that are able to measure the extracellular volume in the heart, which have also been shown to correlate with prognosis in patients with HF and cardiomyopathies [9].

Moreover, a non-negligible number of patients are affected by familial dilated cardiomyopathy (DCM), which can sometimes be easily identified with a simple family pedigree [10]. On this subject, with the advent of next generation sequencing gene techniques, we are now able to identify multiple mutations associated with DCM in more than 50 genes [11]. The most frequent ones are titin (TTN), lamin (LMNA) and desmin (DES). Pathogenic mutations in LMNA [12] and DES [13] as well as filamin C (FLNC) [14] genes are specifically related with frequent arrhythmias and subsequent worse prognosis. Therefore, genetic testing should also be taken into account when stratifying patients, especially because they usually affect young individuals, with less evident HF symptoms in spite of the severe myocardial disease.

The indication for HTx in patients with hypertrophic cardiomyopathy (HCM) is unusual and should be reserved for patients with persistent marked symptoms, after all therapeutic possibilities have been applied, including septal reduction techniques. It is more frequent to perform HTx in patients with HCM with progressive severe left ventricular dysfunction and/or a restrictive pattern.

Arrhythmogenic cardiomyopathy is produced by the alteration of cardiac desmosomes, which predisposes to an abnormal response to mechanical stress. Genetically, it is transmitted predominantly in an autosomal dominant manner with a variable clinical expression and an incomplete penetrance that is dependent of age. It is a frequent cause of sudden death and ventricular arrhythmias, especially in young adults and athletes, because it is linked to severe ventricular arrhythmias, especially when it affects the left ventricle. Furthermore, in spite of the use of implantable cardiac defibrillators (ICD), severe cardiac events including sudden cardiac death and mortality might appear over time, because of progressive biventricular dysfunction and untreatable arrhythmias. Hence, HTx should always be taken into account during follow-up [13, 14].

Restrictive cardiomyopathy (RCM) is the least common and it comprises a group of diseases of the myocardium, characterized by a rigid myocardium that produces diastolic dysfunction that leads to a restrictive physiology, with a normal or reduced systolic and diastolic ventricular volumes and non-thickened or minimally thickened ventricular walls. The majority of the restrictive cardiomyopathies can be secondary to a toxic process (e.g., radiotherapy, hypereosinophilic syndrome, use of anthracyclines), infiltrative disease (e.g., amyloido-sis or sarcoidosis), and storage cardiomyopathy (Anderson-Fabry disease, Danon disease, hemochromatosis) with amyloidosis being the most common etiology. Nonetheless, genetic restrictive cardiomyopathy is also a diagnostic possibility that should be taken into account, especially when family involvement is present. In this regard, DES mutations are charac-terized by severe diastolic dysfunction and atrio-ventricular block, with progressive systolic dysfunction and early-onset end-stage HF, and frequent neuromuscular disease.

In regards to amyloidosis, it is important to distinguish between the different types of amyloid deposit because of the different prognosis and treatment strategies. In immunoglobulin light chain amyloidosis (AL or primary amyloidosis) the evolution of HF is very fast, and although HTx is feasible, significant involvement of other organs should be ruled out. Nonetheless, HTx outcomes are significantly worse, even with bone marrow transplant, and survival rates reach 82% and 65% at 1 and 5 years, respectively [15, 16]. In cases of hereditary transthyretin amyloidosis, HF does not progress as rapidly as in light chain amyloidosis, and it is recom-mended to perform HTx followed by liver transplant at a second time point to prevent further myocardial compromise, although the advent of new drugs to treat transthyretin amyloid and the different mutations involved may change this strategy. In any case, it is also essential to exclude severe amyloid involvement of other organs [17].

Among the different types of cardiomyopathies, serious multi-organ involvement, particu-larly neuromuscular involvement that could compromise the respiratory capacity should always be ruled out. Thus, the decision to go to HTx must be taken after a comprehensive multidisciplinary evaluation that should involve at least, a HF specialist, a pneumologist and a neurologist.

2.3. Functional capacity

Clinical assessment of functional capacity is a subjective measure of the patient's ability to perform daily activities that can easily be obtained, and correlates with the severity of the disease. It is measured by the New York Heart Association (NYHA) scale, which stratifies four groups (functional class) from less to more limitations in physical activity. Candidates for HTx are most of the time in functional class IV despite optimal medical treatment (stage D of the American Heart Association classification), although they can alternate with some periods of partial recovery to functional class III.

In spite of its usefulness, this scale is a subjective measure that an change depending on the patient and physician's interpretation, and should be complemented by the use of more objec-tive tests. The cardiopulmonary exercise test (CPET) measures peak oxygen uptake (VO2), which is the most accurate measure of exercise capacity and cardiopulmonary performance [18]. According to the latest guidelines, a peak VO2 ≤ 14 mL/kg/min or peak VO2 ≤ 12 mL/kg/min in the presence of β-blockers at maximal exertion should be used to include patients in HTx list, although this should not be the unique parameter. In cases of a sub-maximal cardio-pulmonary exercise test, defined as the ratio of carbon dioxide output/oxygen uptake (also called respiratory exchange ratio [RER]) < 1, the use of ventilation to carbon dioxide slope (VE/VCO2) > 35 is also useful because of its prognostic value [19].

Also, the 6-minute walking test (6'WT) measures the distance that the patient is able to walk in 6 minutes and is useful when a cardiopulmonary test is not available. A walking distance of less than 300 m is associated with an annual mortality above 50% [20], and is one of the criteria of AHF.

2.4. Risk scores

Currently, there are several risk scores available that might help in patient stratification, and give support in decision making. In ambulatory patients, there are two risk scores that complement the prognostic information obtained from CPET:

1. The Seattle Heart Failure Model (SHFM) has 21 variables; it is derived from a study of 1125 patients with NYHA class IIIB or IV, during the Prospective Randomized Amlodipine Survival Evaluation (PRAISE) [21]. It was used in the REMATCH trial cohort for predicting 1-year mortality in the medical and LTVAD groups with good accuracy [22]. The model was also prospectively validated in five additional cohorts consisting of 9942 HF patients and 17,307 person-years of follow-up [23]. When an estimated 1-year survival of less than 80% is obtained, patients should be considered for HTx [19].

2. The Heart Failure Survival Score (HFSS) is calculated with the following variables: VO2 max, ejection fraction of the left ventricle, sodium, mean arterial pressure, ischemic etiology, resting heart rate, QRS > 120 ms. Patients in the medium and high risk category should be considered for advanced-HF therapies such as HTx listing or VAD implantation [24].

The Interagency Registry for Mechanically Assisted Circulatory Support (INTERMACS) is a database created in 2006, with information of more than 15,000 patients who received an MCS [25]. The INTERMACS classification was created from this registry and helps to stratify patients in an AHF situation, see **Table 2**. In this regard, patients in a higher INTERMACS profile (1 or 2) seem to have worse post-HTx outcomes than those in better pre-operative condition (INTERMACS 3-4) [26].

2.5. Hemodynamic parameters

Pulmonary hypertension (PHT) is defined by a mean pulmonary arterial pressure greater than 25 mmHg, and usually develops in response to a passive backward transmission of elevated filling pressures from the left ventricle. Nonetheless, irreversible PHT might eventually develop in response to chronic elevated pressures that cause vascular remodeling, and is closely related to primary graft failure (PGF) due to right ventricular failure (RVF), which carries an elevated mortality after HTx [28]. Therefore right heart catheterization is recommended before HTx and should be done periodically, every 3–6 months [19], especially if reversible PHT has been previously confirmed.

The main direct (measured directly during procedure) and indirect (calculated from direct parameters) parameters evaluated during right heart catheterization are:

- Direct parameters: 1-right atrial pressure, 2-sistolic pulmonary arterial pressure (SPAP), 3-mean pulmonary arterial pressure (MPAP), 4-pulmonary capillary wedge pressure (PCWP), and 4-cardiac output (CO).

- Indirect parameters: 1-transpulmonary gradient (TPG): Defined as the difference between mean pulmonary arterial pressure and capillary wedge pressure (TPG = MPAP-PCWP), 2-pulmonary vascular resistance (PVR) defined as TPG/CO is usually expressed in Wood units, 3-cardiac index expressed as the result of CO/body surface area.

Reversible PHT is defined as a drop in SPAP < 50 mmHg, TPG < 12 mmHg and PVR < 3 Woods units after optimization of cardiac index and loading conditions (indicated mainly by central venous pressure, systemic vascular resistance and systemic arterial pressure) by the use of intravenous diuretics, inotropes and vasodilators, if necessary. A combination of inotropes with direct vasodilators (e.g., dobutamine and nitroprusside) and selective vasodilators (e.g., sildenafil, nitric oxide) is also commonly used. It is important to mention that if after the pulmonary vasodilation test the PVR drops <3 UW but the systolic blood pressure falls to less than 85 mmHg, there is still a high risk of PGF after HTx [29, 30].

In any case, but especially when irreversible or fixed PHT is present, it is important to rule out concomitant pulmonary disease, obstructive sleep apnea syndrome or chronic pulmonary

INTERMACS level	Description	1 year survival with LTVAD
1. Cardiogenic Shock ("crash and burn")	Hemodynamic instability with increasing inotropic and vasopressor support, and critical hypoperfusion of target organs.	52.6 ± 5.6%
2. Progressive decline despite inotropic support ("sliding fast" on inotropes)	Dependent on inotropic support but continues with signs of clinical deterioration (worsening renal failure, nutritional depletion, and inability to restore volume balance).	63.1 ± 3.1%
3. Stable but inotrope-dependent ("dependent stability")	Stable with low/intermediate doses of inotropes, but necessary due to arterial hypotension, progressive renal failure, worsening symptoms	78.4 ± 2.5%
4. Resting symptoms on oral therapy ("frequent flyer")	Patient at home on oral therapy but with high doses of diuretics and frequent symptoms of congestion at rest or with regular activity	78.7 ± 3%
5. Exertion intolerant ("housebound")	Comfortable at rest but unable to engage in any activity	93 ± 3.9%
6. Exertion limited ("walking wounded")	Comfortable at rest and without symptoms during daily living activities, but who becomes symptomatic with any meaningful physical exertion	
7. Advanced NYHA class III ("placeholder")	Patient in NYHA class III with no recent episode of acute decompensation	

NYHA: New York Heart Association.

Table 2. INTERMACS patient profile (Source Ponikowsky et al. [27]).

thromboembolism. If there is no responsible pulmonary disease, there are several studies that have shown that the chronic use of bosentan or sildenafil might reduce PHT and acheive reversibility of PHT after 3–4 months of this therapy [31]. If despite an appropriate vasodilator treatment there is no reversibility of the PHT, LTVAD therapy should be considered, together with selective vasodilator treatment (usually sildenafil) [32].

3. Ventricular assist devices as bridge to transplant

MCS has largely evolved over the last years and nowadays it constitutes a real option for patients in AHF situation, especially in those who are in INTERMACS 1 to 4 profiles. As a matter of fact, in 2000, the International Society of Heart and Lung Transplantation (ISHLT) reported that 19.1% of HTxs were mechanically supported, and by the year 2012 this number had increased to 41% [33]. Lately, the clinical outcomes of a Spanish registry of 291 patients supported by STVAD as a BTT strategy have been published, showing an overall survival rate from listing to hospital discharge of 61%, and 1-year survival after listing of 58% [34]. Although there was a significant mortality rate, it is important to mention that the majority of patients were in an emergency situation (INTERMACS 1-2) and were supported by a very heterogeneous group of STVADs. Accordingly, it seems reasonable to use LTVADs as a BTT strategy at an early stage of the disease (INTERMACS 3-4) to improve HTx outcomes.

Irrespective of the design, LTVAD unloads the heart by pumping blood from the left ventricle to the aorta. Technology of LTVADs has been continuously evolving since the creation of the first generation devices, which had a diaphragm and unidirectional valves to replicate the pulsatile cardiac cycle. The HeartMate XVE was approved by the FDA; first as BTT in 1998 and in 2002 as a DT, after the publication of the REMATCH trial. Later advances in technology have been directed to minimize the size of the pump and to increase its durability. Nowadays, continuous flow LTVADs have substituted pulsatile devices; these utilize a permanent magnetic field designed to rapidly spin a single impeller supported by mechanical, hydrodynamic or magnetic bearings. In second-generation continuous flow LTVAD the impeller outflow is directed parallel to the axis of rotation (e.g., Heartmate II, Thoratec and Incor, Berlin Heart) while in the third generation devices the impeller outflow is directed perpendicular to the axis of rotation (e.g., HVAD, Medtronic and HeartMate 3, Abbot). Third generation pumps have lower risk of suction events, more pulsatile waveform, and more precise flow estimation than second-generation pumps, but pump flow has a higher dependency on loading conditions [35].

The best candidates for a BTT strategy are patients in INTERMACS 3-4 profile; especially if a long waiting time for HTx is expected, as it avoids further deterioration, allows clinical optimization, and provides a better quality of life. In this regard, some factors that may increase the difficulty in finding a appropriate donor should be taken into consideration, as for example previous allosensitization or large body size.

BTC LTVAD strategy is the preferred option for those patients with relative contraindications to HTx that could be potentially reversible with hemodynamic support. For instance, most patients with initially irreversible PHT reach reversibility or even normal pulmonary pressure after some months with LTVAD [24]. In a similar fashion, renal dysfunction due to cardiorenal syndrome can improve enough to consider HTx. In this group, we can also include patients with recently diagnosed cancer or obesity (BMI > 35 kg/m^2), in which the implantation of a LTVAD could give them time to re-evaluate candidacy.

Regarding LTVAD as DT, one of the limitations of this strategy is the increase in adverse events associated with long-term use of LTVAD. The ROADMAP study took a sample of 200 patients in INTERMACS 4–7 and divided them into two groups: optimal medical management (OMM) or OMM plus LTVAD. The final result showed an improvement in functional capacity in the second group but with a significant increase in adverse events, especially hemorrhagic complications [36]. Although current indications for DT consider a more advanced profile of patients (criteria derived from the REMATCH and HeartMate II DT trials [37]), the results of the ROADMAP study give us and idea of the advantages and disadvantages of the use of LTVAD as DT, further supporting the fact that HTx remains the ideal therapy in this population.

Regardless of the selected strategy, the most important fact is to ensure a correct selection of candidates for LTVAD implantation. One of the tools used to predict outcomes of these patients using mechanical support is the HeartMate II Risk Score, which is derived from an analysis of the HeartMate II registry. Briefly, it is based on five variables (age, serum albumin, creatinine, INR, and center volume of LVAD) used to create an equation that predicts mortality at 90 days [38]. Moreover, because LTVADs only support the left ventricle, one of the critical points to take into consideration is the potential right ventricular failure (RVF) after MCS is initiated. Nowadays, there are no comprehensively evaluated tools to predict RVF, but some hemodynamic and echocardiographic parameters might be useful. Concerning hemodynamic evaluation, a right ventricular stroke work index less than 250 mmHg·mLm^2 [39], right atrial pressure > 15 mmHg and central venous pressure/PCWP >0.63 are considered important risk factors of RVF [40]. Echocardiographic parameters include tricuspid annular motion (TAPSE) < 7.5 mm [41], right ventricular to left ventricular end diastolic diameter ratio > 0.72 [42], severe tricuspid regurgitation, right ventricular short/long axis ratio > 0.6 [43] and right ventricular free wall strain [44]. A biventricular approach using continuous blood flow pumps has recently been reported with limited success considering the significant number of adverse events during follow-up [45].

Finally, it is very important to ensure optimal patient's self-care training by specialized nurses, and appropriate follow-up is indispensable for the success of a LTVAD program. Daily care of the device, especially considering the correct management of the driveline wound is of paramount importance to avoid infection. Moreover, the correct management of concomitant cardiovascular risk factors such as hypertension or diabetes, and other comorbidities is also a relevant issue in these patients that should be pursued.

4. Inclusion in heart transplant waiting list

The decision of including a patient in the HTx waiting list is not easy and should be taken together by a medical and surgical team, in a case-by-case comprehensive evaluation. Only stage D HF patients without any other treatment option should be evaluated for HTx, because of the shortage of organs, the intrinsic risk of surgery, and the risk of rejection and complications due to immunosuppressant therapy. **Table 3** shows the indications for HTx.

Therefore, it is important to undergo an exhaustive study of the patient before listing for HTx, in order to exclude any significant risk factor that might compromise outcomes after HTx. Last but not least, the patient must be motivated, well informed and in an optimal psychological state to follow the intensive pharmacologic treatment that follows the HTx. **Table 4** shows recommended studies that should be done when evaluating candidacy for HTx.

To conclude, patients with LTVAD as BTC can be included in the waiting list once reversible PHT is confirmed by a right heart catheterization, and/or there is significant improvement in renal function (glomerular filtration rate [GFR] > 30 cc/min/1.73 m^2, especially if there is no evidence of intrinsic renal damage: absence of significant proteinuria without significant abnormalities in renal ultrasonography), and other parameters. In patients with concomitant treated malignant neoplasm, a thoughtful evaluation tackling life expectancy and relapse possibilities, together with an oncologist's evaluation should be performed before listing for HTx.

Absolute Indications

1. Hemodynamic compromise due to HF

· Refractory cardiogenic shock

· Documented dependence on IV inotropic support to maintain adequate organ perfusion

2. Peak VO2 less than 14 mL per kg per minute with achievement of anaerobic metabolism or less than 12 mL per kg per minute with the use of β-blockers

3. Severe symptoms of ischemia that consistently limit routine activity and are not amenable to coronary artery bypass surgery or percutaneous coronary intervention

4. Recurrent symptomatic ventricular arrhythmias refractory to all therapeutic modalities

Relative Indications

1. In the presence of sub-maximal cardiopulmonary exercise test (RER<1.05), ventilation equivalent of carbon dioxide (VE/VCO2) slope > 35

2. Use of prognostic scores in conjunction with cardiopulmonary exercise stress test. A 1-year estimated survival calculated by the SHFM less than 80% and a HFSS in high/medium risk range

3. Recurrent unstable ischemia not amenable to other intervention

4. Recurrent instability of fluid balance/renal function not due to patient noncompliance with medical regimen

Insufficient indications

1. Low left ventricular ejection fraction

2. History of NYHA functional class III or IV symptoms of HF

3. Peak VO2 greater than 15 mL per kg per minute (and greater than 55% predicted) without other indications

---

V02: Oxygen consumption; SHFM: Seattle Heart Failure Model; HFFS: Heart Failure Survival Score; NYHA: New York Heart Association.

Table 3. Heart transplant indications (Source Kirklin JK et al. and Hunt S et al. [46, 19]).

- Clinical history and complete physical examination
- Size/weight/body mass index
- Blood Typing and Immune suitability study
· ABO blood group
· HLA typing
· Panel-reactive antibody (PRA)
· Flow cytometry (Luminex)
- Assessment of severity of cardiac insufficiency
- Multiple organ function evaluation
· General analysis with glycemia, lipid profile, renal function, hepatic profile, coagulation, thyroid hormones, natriuretic peptides
· First-hour urinalysis with proteinuria
· Chest x-ray
· Functional respiratory tests with arterial gases
· Abdominal ultrasound or thoraco-abdominal CT scan
· Doppler echo of supra-aortic trunks (if more than 50 years, diabetic, ischemic cardiomyopathy or clinical suspicion)
· Lower extremity ankle/arm or Doppler echo index (if more than 50 years, diabetic, ischemic cardiomyopathy or clinical suspicion)
· Electroencephalogram
· Bone densitometry (if more than 50 years, woman or clinical suspicion)

- Infectious assessment
· Hepatitis B virus: surface antigen, antibody of surface, anti-core
· Antibody hepatitis C virus
· Antibody hepatitis A virus
· Human immunodeficiency virus
· VDRL (venereal disease research laboratory)
· Herpes Simplex antibody
· Cytomegalovirus antibody
· Toxoplasma antibody
· Epstein–Barr antibody
· Varicella antibody

· Tuberculin or quantiferon test
- Vaccination
· Influenza (annual)
· Hepatitis B and A if it has not been done
· Pneumococcal vaccine (every 5 years)
- Study of hidden malignant neoplasm
· Fecal occult blood test × 3
· Colonoscopy (if >50 years old)
· Mammography (if indicated or > 40 years)
· Gynecological examination and vaginal cytology (if >18 years old and sexually active)
· Specific prostate antigen and rectal examination (men >50 years old)
- Other evaluations
· Social worker
· Psychiatry
· Psychosocial and economic assessment

HLA: human leucocyte antigen and CT: computerized tomography.

Table 4. Recommended studies in the evaluation of candidates for HTx. Adapted from Mehra et al. [29].

4.1. Immune suitability evaluation

Screening for humoral rejection is done through the panel-reactive antibody (PRA) test, which determines the presence of circulating anti-HLA antibodies. With this cytotoxic test, it is possible to estimate the sensitization of the recipient by the percentage of the serum reactivity that activates complement against a panel of the most common HLAs in the recipient's country. A PRA > 10% is considered positive and is a relative contraindication for HTx. In these cases, it is recommended to perform a prospective cross-match between the lymphocytes of the donor and recipient's serum before HTx. Currently, it is also possible to identify and quantify the amount of antibodies against surface HLA antigens using a flow cytometry immunofluorescence technique. This method (Luminex) is much more sensitive than the PRA and allows a better assessment of the risk of positive cross-reactivity at the time of HTx and eventual humoral rejection.

Patients can be sensitized after pregnancies, blood transfusions, after previous transplantation or after the implant of a ventricular assist device, although sometimes there is no obvious sensitizer event, and it is thought to be due to cross-reactivity between bacterial or viral epitopes and HLAs. In case that the recipient has a ventricular assist device, it is recommended to repeat the PRA and flow cytometry every 2–3 months. If blood transfusions are required, the PRA and flow cytometry should be repeated 2 weeks after the transfusion and each month during 6 months [29].

The presence of anti-HLA antibodies with high levels of median fluorescent intensity or MFI (units used to quantify antibodies), usually over 3000–5000, depending on the immunology laboratory, is considered potentially cytotoxic. By this technique it is also possible to obtain a calculated PRA (cPRA), which gives the percentage of unacceptable HLAs in the donor population. For example, if the cPRA is 80%, it means that only 20% of all possible donors in this specific population will be compatible with the receptor. Although the cPRA cut-points are not clearly established, some authors consider an absolute contraindication if cPRA is above 50–70%, and thus recommend a desensitization therapy before HTx [47]. In these cases it is also necessary to perform a virtual cross-match at the time of HTx, consisting of the evaluation of anti-HLA receptor antibodies titters relative to the donor HLA. If the virtual cross-match is positive, the risk of hyperacute rejection is very high and the donor organ must not be accepted.

5. Infectious evaluation and vaccination

A complete serologic status of the potential recipient should always be obtained before HTx, especially considering previous exposure to cytomegalovirus and Mycobacterium tuberculosis, as it is crucial when defining infectious prophylaxis after HTx.

The human immunodeficiency virus infection with undetectable viral load is not a contraindication to HTx at present, although each case must be assessed individually and retroviral treatment should be adapted to avoid interference with calcineurin inhibitors [48].

Patients with chronic hepatitis B infection (defined by the presence of hepatitis B surface antigen) have equal survival rates compared to the rest of the cohort, unless there is significant liver disease. In this setting, liver cirrhosis should be ruled out with biopsy if necessary, and antivirals should be given in order to lower viral load, since there is a risk of reactivation of the disease with immunosuppression after HTx. Similarly, when hepatitis C virus serology is positive, the quantitative viral load and degree of liver disease must be determined. If circulating HCV is detected, the disease is active and antiviral treatment must be prescribed to eliminate the virus. An altered hepatic function, which is not justified by HF, or a liver biopsy with evidence of cirrhosis, should be considered an absolute contraindication [30].

Finally, vaccination against hepatitis A and B viruses is also recommended if not previously given, as well as vaccination against Pneumococcus (every 5 years), Influenza (annual) and *Haemophilus influenzae* before the HTx [29].

6. Risk factors and contraindications

Absolute contraindications for HTx are progressively diminishing because of the improved treatment strategies both for comorbidities and immunosuppressive therapies after HTx, so nowadays it is preferable to talk about risk factors that increase post-HTx morbidity and mortality than contraindications. According to the latest recommendations from the ISHLT [19] the most important HTx risk factors are classified in **Table 5**. Nonetheless, it is important to especially consider the following:

- Patients with age > 70 years could be considered for HTx based on individual evaluation. It is important to take into consideration that this population has lower rates of rejection but higher mortality than younger patients.

- Patients with a body mass index (BMI) > 35 kg/m^2 should wait until they achieve a BMI ≤ 35 kg/m^2 to be included in the waiting list, because patients with BMI > 35 kg/m^2 have more difficulty in finding an adequate donor. Besides, there is some evidence that this group of patients have an increase in post-operative morbidity and mortality.

- Poorly controlled diabetes (glycosylated hemoglobin [HbA1c] >7.5% or 58 mmol/mol) with end-organ damage (other than non-proliferative retinopathy) is a relative contraindication for HTx.

- Presence of irreversible renal dysfunction with GFR <30 cc/min/1.73 m^2 should be considered a relative contraindication for HTx alone, although the combination of heart and kidney transplant could be considered.

- Clinically severe symptomatic cerebrovascular disease could be considered a contraindication for HTx based on the existence of a study that shows how these patients have an increased risk of stroke and functional decline as an independent variable after transplantation [49]. Peripheral vascular disease that limits rehabilitation without possibility of re-vascularization continues to be a contraindication.

- Frailty defined as a clinically identifiable disorder of amplified vulnerability of age-related decline in reserve and function across multiple physiologic systems brought on with minor stressors [50] should be assessed before HTx, the presence of three of five possible symptoms, including unintentional weight loss of 5 kg within the past year, muscle loss, fatigue, slow walking speed and low levels of physical activity define a fragile patient.

- Psychosocial evaluation previous to HTx is important in order to make sure that the patient is going to be able to accomplish an optimal care after transplantation. Absence of this condition is considered a relative contraindication.

Absolute contraindications

- Systemic disease with life expectancy <2 years:

· Active neoplasm (if preexisting, evaluation with an oncology specialist is necessary to stratify the risk of recurrence and establish a time to wait after remission)

· Systemic disease with multi-organ involvement (systemic lupus erythematosus, amyloidosis, sarcoidosis)

· Severe chronic obstructive pulmonary disease ($FEV_1 < 1$ L)

· Renal or hepatic severe dysfunction, if associated renal or liver transplant is not performed

- Irreversible pulmonary hypertension

· Pulmonary artery systolic pressure > 50 mmHg

· Transpulmonary gradient >12 mmHg

· Pulmonary vascular resistance >3 Wood units despite treatment

Relative contraindications

- Age > 70 years (carefully selected patients may be considered)

- Diabetes with end-organ damage (except non-proliferative retinopathy) or persistent poor glycemic control (HbA1c > 7.5%) despite treatment

- Active infection, except VAD infection. Patients with HIV, hepatitis, Chagas disease and tuberculosis can be considered with strict management

- Severe peripheral arterial or cerebrovascular disease not suitable for treatment

- Other serious comorbidities with poor prognosis, such as neuromuscular diseases

- Obesity: BMI > 35 kg/m²

- Cachexia: BMI < 18 kg/m²

- Frailty: when three of five possible symptoms (including unintentional weight loss of >5 kg within the past year, muscle loss, fatigue, slow walking speed, and low levels of physical activity) are present

- Current tobacco, alcohol or drug abuse

- Insufficient social support

- Elevated panel-reactive antibody test defined as >10%

FEV_1: forced expiratory volume in 1 s; VAD: ventricular assist device; HIV: human immunodeficiency virus; BMI: body mass index.

Table 5. Contraindications for heart transplant (Source Sanchez-Enrique et al. [51]).

7. Heart transplantation waiting list priority

Nearly 100,000 people worldwide have received a new heart since the first HTx 50 years ago, 8000 of them in Spain, which makes it a country with a remarkable experience [52]. Each year priority criteria on the waiting list are reviewed. The 2017 priority criteria in adult population in Spain are summarized in **Table 6**.

The objective of this model is to prioritize those patients in the most critical situation. The ASIS-TC study showed a median waiting time for patients in urgency Grade 0 of 7.6 days allowing HTx in nearly 80% of this population [34]. Other countries like the U.S have a more heterogeneous group of patients listed in emergency situation (Status 1A) (**Table 7**), which makes waiting times more prolonged, between 47 and 413 days, depending on the region

Urgency Grade 0: national (priority over the rest of grades**)**

- Patients with STVAD of complete support[a].

- Patients with extracorporeal membrane oxygenation (ECMO) or partial support STVAD for at least 48 hours if there is no evidence of multi-organ failure[b,c].

- Patients with dysfunctional LTVAD[d] secondary to mechanical dysfunction or thromboembolism.

Urgency Grade 1: regional (priority over elective patients in reference zone**)**

- Patients with a normally functioning external LTVAD[e].

- Patients with dysfunctional LTVAD secondary to driveline infection, gastrointestinal bleeding or right heart failure.

Elective

- Patients not included in Grade 0 or Grade 1 categories.

STVAD: short-term ventricular assist device; LTVAD: long-term ventricular assist device.[a]e.g., Levitronix Centrimag.
[b]e.g., Impella CP, Impella 5.0, Tandem Heart.
[c]Maximum time in urgency Grade 0 will be 7 days, once this time has passed the patient will be in Urgency Grade 1.
[d]e.g., BerlinHeart Excor, Hearmate II, Heartmate 3, Heartware HVAD.
[e]e.g., BerlinHeart Excor.

Table 6. Priority criteria for heart transplant donors in Spain (Adapted from barge et al. [53]).

[47]. This shows the importance of defining homogeneous criteria to define each stage of classification for HTx waiting list, especially in the setting of emergency. A new more precise classification for the U.S. is expected to be published in 2018.

Status code	Criteria
Status 1A	• ECMO
	• IABP
	• Inpatient TAH
	• Mechanical ventilation
	• Continuous infusion of a single high-dose intravenous inotrope or multiple intravenous inotropes, and with continuous hemodynamic monitoring of left ventricular filling pressures
	• LVAD, RVAD, or BiVAD for 30 days
	• Mechanical circulatory support with significant device-related complications (thromboembolism, device infection, mechanical failure, or life threatening ventricular arrhythmias)
Status 1B	• Uncomplicated LVAD, RVAD, BiVAD after 30 days have been used.
	• Outpatient TAH
	• Continuous infusion of intravenous inotropes
Status 2	• Candidates not meeting 1A or 1B criteria
Status 7	• Temporarily inactive, most often due to infection

BiVAD: biventricular assist device; ECMO: extracorporeal membrane oxygenation; IABP: intra-aortic balloon pump; LVAD: left ventricular assist device; RVAD: right ventricular assist device; TAH: total artificial heart.

Table 7. Status codes for heart transplantation in U.S. (Source Kittleson et al. [47]).

8. Conclusions

Cardiovascular diseases are the main cause of death around the world, and with the improvement in therapeutics leading to an increase of life expectancy it is probable that we will see increasing number of patients with HF. Also, prevalence of HF in the overall population ranges between 1 and 2% depending on the country. Therefore it is expected that the number of patients with AHF will continue rising after this review. Yet it is important keep in mind some concepts:

- Establishing HF etiology could play a key role in the management and prognosis of the patient and his family, especially if there is an identified genetic cardiomyopathy.

- NYHA scale is useful to determine functional capacity, however objective tests should be used in order to establish a more reliable prognosis in this population.

- Optimization of HF treatment with medication and devices according to the latest guidelines is mandatory before considering advanced therapies.

- LTVADs as BTT or BTC is an appropriate management strategy in selected cases, especially if they are in an INTERMACS 3 profile.

- HTx remains the optimal therapy for patients in stage D HF, however with the shortage of donors and the improvement in technology, LTVADs as DT might change the management strategy in developed countries.

Acknowledgements

We would like to thank Dr. Nicolás Manito and Dr. Josep Roca for their advice, tireless teaching and wisdom. Also Magda Nebot, Laia Rosenfeld and Carmen Mejuto for their invaluable daily work and support.

Conflict of interest

We declare no conflicts of interest in writing this chapter.

Appendices and nomenclature

HTx: heart transplant

HF: heart failure

AHF: advanced heart failure

CS: cardiogenic shock

VAD: ventricular assist device

MCS: mechanical circulatory support

BTT: bridge to transplant

BTC: bridge to candidacy

BTD: bridge to decision

STVAD: short-term ventricular assist device

LTVAD: long-term ventricular assist device

BTR: bridge to recovery

DT: destination therapy

NYHA: New York heart association

PCWP: pulmonary capillary wedge pressure

RAP: right atrial pressure

DCM: dilated cardiomyopathy

HCM: hypertrophic cardiomyopathy

RCM: restrictive cardiomyopathy

CPET: cardiopulmonary exercise testing

VO2: oxygen uptake

VE/VC02: ventilation to carbon dioxide slope

RER: respiratory exchange ratio

6'WT: 6-minute walking test

SHFM: Seattle Heart Failure Model

HFSS: heart failure survival score

INTERMACS: Interagency Registry for Mechanically Assisted Circulatory Support

PHT: pulmonary hypertension

PGF: primary graft failure

RVF: right ventricular failure

SPAP: systolic pulmonary arterial pressure

MPAP: mean pulmonary arterial pressure

CO: cardiac output

TPG: transpulmonary gradient

PVR: pulmonary vascular resistance

ISHLT: International Society of Heart and Lung Transplantation

BMI: body mass index

HLA: human leucocyte antigen

PRA: panel-reactive antibody

BiVAD: biventricular assist device

ECMO: extracorporeal membrane oxygenation

IABP: intra-aortic balloon pump

LVAD: left ventricular assist device

RVAD: right ventricular assist device

TAH: total artificial heart

Author details

Ulises López-Cardoza, Carles Díez-López and José González-Costello*

*Address all correspondence to: jgonzalez@bellvitgehospital.cat

Advanced Heart Failure and Transplant Unit, Heart Disease Institute, Hospital Universitari de Bellvitge, IDIBELL, L'Hospitalet de Llobregat, Barcelona, Spain

References

[1] McMurray JJ, Adamopoulos S, Anker SD, et al. ESC guidelines for the diagnosis and treatment of acute and chronic heart failure 2012 of the European society of cardiology. Developed in collaboration with the heart failure association (HFA) of the ESC. European Heart Journal. 2012;**14**:803-869. DOI: 10.1093/eurjhf/hfs105

[2] Metra M, Ponikowski P, Dickstein K, et al. Advanced chronic heart failure: A position statement from the study group on advanced heart failure of the heart failure Association of the European Society of cardiology. European Journal of Heart Failure. 2007;**9**:684-694. DOI: 10.1016/j.ejheart.2007.04.003

[3] Zannad F, McMurray JJ, Krum H, et al. Eplerenone in patiens with systolic heat failure and mild symtoms. The New England Journal of Medicine. 2011;**364**:11-21. DOI: 10.1056/NEJMoa1009492

[4] Jhund PS, Macintyre K, Simpson CR, et al. Long-term trends in first hospitalization for heart failure and subsequent survival between 1986 and 2003: A population study of 5.1 million people. Circulation. 2009;**119**:515-523. DOI: 10.1161/CIRCULATIONAHA. 108.812172

[5] González-Vílchez F, Gómez-Bueno M, Almenar-Bonet L, et al. Registro español de trasplante Cardiaco. XXVIII Informe Oficial de la Sección de Insuficiencia Cardiaca de la Sociedad Española de Cardiología (1984-2016). Revista Española de Cardiología. 2017;**70**:1098-1109. DOI: 10.106/j.recesp.2017.07.032

[6] Setoguchi S, Stevenson LW, Schneewelss S. Repeated hospitalizations predict mortality in the community population with heart failure. American Heart Journal. 2007;**154**:260-266. DOI: 10.1016/j.ahj.2007.01.041

[7] Roig-Minguell E, Pérez-Villa F, Castel-Lavilla MA. Estudio y selección del receptor de trasplante cardiaco. In: Trasplante cardiaco. 1st ed. Pulpon LA, Crespo Leiro MG, editors. Buenos Aires: Editorial Médica Panamericana; 2009. 15-30 p

[8] Gulati A, Jabbour A, Ismali TF, et al. Association of fibrosis with mortality and sudden cardiac death in patients with nonischemic dilated cardiomyopathy. Journal of the American Medical Association. 2013;**309**:896-908. DOI: 10.1001/jama.2013.1363

[9] Radenkovic D, Weingärtner S, Ricketts L. T1 mapping in cardiac MRI. Heart Failure Reviews. 2017;**22**:415-430. DOI: 10.1007/s10741-017-9627-2

[10] Pinto YM et al. Proposal for a revised definition of dilated cardiomyopathy, hypokinetic non-dilated cardiomyopathy, and its implications for clinical practice: A position statement of the ESC working group on myocardial and pericardial diseases. European Heart Journal. 2016;**14**-37(23):1850-1858. DOI: 10.1093/eurheartj/ehv727. Epub 2016 Jan 19

[11] Hershberger RE, Morales A, Siegfried JD. Clinical and genetic issues in dilated cardiomyopathy: A review for genetics professionals. Genetics in Medicine. 2010;**12**:655-667. DOI: 10.1097/GIM.0b013e3181f2481f

[12] Captur G et al. Lamin and Heart. Heart. 2018;**104**(6):468-479. DOI: 10.1136/heartjnl-2017-312338

[13] Bermúdez-Jiménez FJ, et al. The novel desmin mutation p.Glu401Asp impairs filament formation, disrupts cell membrane integrity and causes severe arrhythmogenic left ventricular cardiomyopathy/dysplasia. Circulation. 2017;**137**(15):1595-1610. DOI: 10.1161/CIRCULATIONAHA.117.028719

[14] Ortiz-Genga MF et al. Truncating FLNC mutations are associated with high-risk dilated and arrhythmogenic cardiomyopathies. Journal of the American College of Cardiology. 2016;**68**(22):2440-2451. DOI: 10.1016/j.jacc.2016.09.927

[15] Roig E, Almenar L, González-Vílchez F, et al. Outcomes of heart transplantation for cardiac amyloidosis: Subanalysis of the spanish registry for heart transplantation. American Journal of Transplantation. 2009;**9**:1414-1419. DOI: 10.1111/j.1600-6143.2009.02643.x

[16] Arvidsson S, Pilebro B, Westermark P, et al. Amyloid cardiomyopathy in hereditary transthyretin V30M amyloidosis—Impact of sex and amyloid fibril composition. PLoS One. 2015;**10**:e0143456. DOI: 10.1371/journal.pone.0143456

[17] Lladó L, Fabregat J, Ramos E, Balletas C, Roca J, Casasnovas C. Sequential heart and liver transplantation for familial amyloid polyneuropathy. Medicina Clínica (Barcelona). 2014;**142**:211-214. DOI: 10.1016/j.medcli.2013.10.022

[18] Balady GJ, Morise AP. Mann DL, Exercise testing. In: Zipes DP, Libby P, Bonow RO, editors. Braunwald's Heart Disease: A Textbook of Cardiovascular Medicine. 10th ed. Philadelphia: Elsevier Saunders; 2015. p. 159

[19] Mehra MR, Canter CE, Hannan MM, et al. The 2016 International Society for Heart Lung Transplantation: A 10 year update. The Journal of Heart and Lung Transplantation. 2016;**35**:1-23. DOI: 10.1016/j.healun.2015.10.023

[20] Zugck C, Kruger C, Durr S, et al. Is the 6-minute walk test a reliable substitute for peak oxygen uptake in patients with dilated cardiomyopathy? European Heart Journal. 2000;**21**:540-549. DOI: 10.1053/euhj.1999.1861

[21] Pfeffer MA, Skali H. PRAISE (prospective randomized amlodipine survival evaluation) and criticism. JACC Heart Fail. 2013;**1**:315-317. DOI: 10.1016/j.jchf.2013.05.005

[22] Levy WC, Mozaffarian D, Linker DT, et al. Can the Seattle heart failure model be used to risk-stratify heart failure patients for potential left ventricular assist device therapy? Journal of Heart Lung Transplant. 2009;**28**:231-236. DOI: 10.1016/j.healun.2008.12.015

[23] Seattle Heart Failure Model. University of Washington [Internet]. 2107. Available from: https://depts.washington.edu/shfm/ [Accessed 2017-12-14]

[24] Mikus E, Stepanenko A, Krabatsch T, et al. Reversibility of fixed pulmonary hypertension in left ventricular assist device support recipients. European Journal of Cardio-Thoracic Surgery. 2011;**40**:971-977. DOI: 10-1016/j.ejcts.2011.01.019

[25] Kirklin JK, Naftel DC, Pagani FD, et al. Seventh INTERMACS annual report: 15000 patients and counting. The Journal of Heart and Lung Transplantation. 2015;**34**:1495-1504. DOI: 10.1016/j.healun.2015.10.003

[26] Fonarow GC, Adams KF, Abraham WT, et al. Risk stratification for in-hospital mortality in acutely decompensated heart failure: Classification and regression tree analysis. Journal of the American Medical Association. 2005;**293**:572-580. DOI: 10.1001/jama.293.5.572

[27] Ponikowski P, Voors AA, Anker SD, et al. ESC guidelines for the diagnosis and treatment of acute and chronic heart failure: The task force for the diagnosis and treatment of

acute and chronic heart failure of the European Society of Cardiology (ESC).Developed with the special contribution of the heart failure association (HFA) of the ESC. European Journal of Heart Failure. 2016;**18**. 2016:891-975. DOI: 0.1002/ejhf.592

[28] Rodríguez-Padial L, Escribano P, Lázaro M, et al. Comments on the 2015 ESC/ERS guidelines for the diagnosis and treatment of pulmonary hypertension. Revista Española de Cardiología. 2016;**69**:102-108. DOI: 10.1016/j.rec.2015.11.030

[29] Mehra MR, Kobashigawa J, Starling R, et al. Listing criteria for heart transplantation: International Society for Heart and Lung Transplantation guidelines for the care of cardiac transplant candidates, 2006. Journal of Heart Lung Transplant. 2006;**25**:1024-1042. DOI: 10.1016/j.healun.2006.06.008

[30] Crespo-Leiro MG, Almenar-Bonet L, Alonso-Pulpon L, et al. Conferencia de consenso de los grupos españoles de trasplante cardiaco. Revista Española de Cardiología. 2007;**7**:4B-54B. DOI: 10.1016/S1131-3587(07)75240-8

[31] Pons J, Leblanc MH, Bernier M, et al. Effects of chronic sildenafil use on pulmonary hemodynamics and clinical outcomes in heart transplantation. The Journal of Heart and Lung Transplantation. 2012;**31**:1281-1287. DOI: 10.1016/j.healun.2012.09.009

[32] Tedford RJ, Hemnes AR, Russell SD, et al. PDE5A inhibitor treatment of persistent pulmonary hypertension after mechanical circulatory support. Circulation. Heart Failure. 2008;**1**:213-219. DOI: 10.1161/CIRCHEARTFAILURE.108.796789

[33] Stehlik J, Edwards LB, Kucheryavaya AY, et al. The registry of the International Society for Heart and Lung Transplantation: Twenty-eighth adult heart transplant report—2011. The Journal of Heart and Lung Transplantation. 2011;**30**:1078-1094. DOI: 10.1016/j. healun.2011.08.003

[34] Barge-Caballero E, Almenar-Bonet L, González-Vílchez F, et al. Clinical outcomes of temporary mechanical circulatory support as a direct bridge to heart transplantation: A nationwide Spanish registry. European Journal of Heart Failure. 2018;**20**(1):178-186. DOI: 10.1002/EJHF.956

[35] Mancini D, Colombo PC. Left ventricular assist devices: A rapidly evolving alternative to transplant. Journal of the American College of Cardiology. 2015;**65**:2542-2555. DOI: 10.1016/j.jacc.2015.04.039

[36] Estep JD, Starling RC, Hormanshof DA, et al. Risk assessment and comparative effectiveness of left ventricular assist device and medical management in ambulatory heart failure patients: Results from the ROADMAP study. Journal of the American College of Cardiology. 2015;**66**:1747-1761. DOI: 10.1016/j.jacc.2015.07.075

[37] Slaughter MS, Rogers JG, Milano CA, et al. Advanced heart failure treated with continuous-flow left ventricular assist device. The New England Journal of Medicine. 2009;**361**:2241-2251. DOI: 10.1056/NEJMoa0909938

[38] Cowger J, Sundareswaran K, Rogers JG, et al. Predicting survival in patients receiving continuous flow left ventricular assist devices: the HeartMate II risk score. Journal of the American College of Cardiology. 2013;**61**:313-321. DOI: 10.1016/j.jacc.2012.09.055

[39] Fitzpatrick JR 3rd, Frederick JR, Hsu VM, et al. Risk score derived from pre-operative data analysis predicts the need for biventricular mechanical circulatory support. The Journal of Heart and Lung Transplantation 2008;**27**:1286-1292. DOI: 10.1016/j.healun.2008.09.006

[40] Kormos RL, Teuteberg JJ, Pagani FD, et al. Right ventricular failure in patients with the HeartMate II continuous-flow left ventricular assist device: Incidence, risk factors, and effect on outcomes. The Journal of Thoracic and Cardiovascular Surgery. 2010;**139**:1316-1324. DOI: 10.1016/j.jtcvs.2009.11.020

[41] Puwanant S, Hamilton KK, Klodell CT, et al. Tricuspid annular motion as a predictor of severe right ventricular failure after left ventricular assist device implantation. The Journal of Heart and Lung Transplantation. 2008;**27**:1102-1107. DOI: 10.1016/j.healun. 2008.07.022

[42] Vivo RP, Cordero-Reyes AM, Qamar U, et al. Increased right to left ventricle diameter ratio is a strong predictor of right ventricular failure after left ventricular assist device. The Journal of Heart and Lung Transplantation. 2013;**32**:792-799. DOI: 10.1016/j. healun.2013.05.016

[43] Potapov E, Stepanenko A, Dandel M, et al. Tricuspid in competence and geometry of the right ventricle as predictor so fright ventricular function after implantation of a left ventricular assist device. The Journal of Heart and Lung Transplantation. 2008;**27**:1275-1281. DOI: 10.1016/j.healun.2008.08.012

[44] Cameli M, Lisi M, Righini FM, et al. Speckle tracking echocardiography as a new technique to evaluate right ventricular function in patients with left ventricular assist device therapy. The Journal of Heart and Lung Transplantation. 2013;**32**:424-430. DOI: 10.1016/j. healun.2012.12.010

[45] Arabía FA et al. Biventricular support with intracorporeal continuous flow centrifugal ventricular assist devices. The Annals of Thoracic Surgery. 2018;**105**(2):548-555. DOI: 10.1016/j.athoracsur.2017.08.019

[46] Yancy CW, Jessup M, Bozkurt B. 2013 ACCF/AHA guideline for the management of heart failure: A report of the American College of Cardiology Foundation/American Heart Association Task Force on Practice Guidelines. Journal of the American College of Cardiology. 2013 Oct 15;**62**(16):e147-e239. DOI: 0.1016/j.jacc.2013.05.019. Epub 2013 Jun 5

[47] Kittleson M, Kobashigawa JA. Cardiac transplantation: Current outcomes and contemporary controversies. JACC Heart Fail. 2017;**5**:857-868. DOI: 10.1016/j.jchf.2017.08.021

[48] Uriel N, Jorde UP, Cotarlan V, et al. Heart transplantation in human immunodeficiency virus-positive patients. The Journal of Heart and Lung Transplantation. 2009;**28**:667-669. DOI: 10.1016/J.HEALUN.2009.04.005

[49] Patlolla V, Mogulla V, DeNofrio D, et al. Outcomes in patients with symptomatic cerebrovascular disease undergoing heart transplantation. Journal of the American College of Cardiology. 2011;**58**:1036-1041. DOI: 10.1016/j.jacc.2011.04.038

[50] Clegg A, Young J, Iliffe S, et al. Frailty in elderly people. Lancet. 2013;**381**:752-762. DOI: 10.1016/S0140-6736(12)62167-9

[51] Sánchez-Enrique C, Jorde UP, González-Costello J. Heart transplant and mechanical circulatory support in patients with advanced heart failure. Revista Española de Cardiología. 2017;**70**:371-381. DOI: 10.1016/j.rec2016.12.036

[52] González-Vílchez F, Gómez-Bueno M, Almenar-Bonet L, et al. Registro español de trasplante cardiaco. XXVIII Informe Oficial de la Sección de Insuficiencia Cardiaca de la Sociedad Española de Cardiología (1984-2016). In: Revista Española de Cardiología. 2017;**70**(12):1098-1109. DOI: 10.106/j.recesp.2017.07.032

[53] Barge-Caballero E, González-Vílchez F, Farrero-Torres M, Segovia-Cubero J. Selección de lo mejor del año 2017 en trasplante cardiaco y asistencia ventricular. Revista Española de Cardiología. 2018;**71**(4):300-301. DOI: 10.1016/j.recesp.2017.10.011

5

Cardiac Re-Transplantation: A Growing Indication with Unique Considerations

Robert JH Miller and Kiran Khush

Abstract

Cardiac re-transplantation (ReTx) accounts for a small proportion of the patients undergoing heart transplantation every year. However, due to improved patient management following transplant, the number of patients potentially requiring re-transplant is growing. We will review the current epidemiology of ReTx and describe the potential increase in candidates for ReTx. We will also highlight important characteristics of patients undergoing ReTx including co-morbidities and allosensitization. We will summarize single-center and registry data on patient outcomes following ReTx, and discuss patient selection. Finally, we will outline the management of patients following cardiac ReTx as well as alternate therapies and ethical considerations in cardiac ReTx.

Keywords: cardiac Retransplantation, epidemiology, outcomes

1. Introduction

There are over 5000 heart transplants performed annually worldwide. Survival following cardiac transplantation has improved dramatically, with one-year survival approaching 85% with a median survival of 11 years [1]. As a result, many patients are now surviving to develop late complications of cardiac transplantation such as chronic rejection, cardiac allograft vasculopathy (CAV), or late graft failure. Unfortunately, there are few medical therapies that significantly alter the development and progression of these complications, particularly at advanced stages [2, 3]. Cardiac retransplantation (ReTx) offers possible benefit to patients who survive to develop these late complications, particularly those patients who have developed left ventricular systolic dysfunction [4].

The first ReTx was performed in 1974 at Stanford, and the first group of patients was reported in 1977 by Copeland et al., which included 5 patients who underwent ReTx for either CAV or acute graft failure. ReTx currently comprises 3.0% of adult cardiac transplants [3, 5, 6], and a similar proportion of pediatric transplants [7]. While this proportion may seem small, it mirrors the proportion of patients transplanted for congenital heart disease, hypertrophic cardiomy-opathy, restrictive cardiomyopathy, and valvulvar cardiomyopathy [5]. Additionally, as more patients survive to develop late complications, the number of patients who are candidates for ReTx will rise. Given this increase, ReTx will potentially outgrow these other indications for cardiac transplant.

2. Epidemiology of cardiac re-transplantation

The number of patients undergoing ReTx has been gradually increasing over time. Between 2000 and 2005, ReTx accounted for 2.9% of all heart transplants [3]. Between January 2009 and June 2015 there were 722 patients who underwent ReTx, which constituted 3.1% of heart transplants. While this seems like a small increase over time, there has been a simultaneous shift towards more rigorous patient selection for ReTx. This shift has been a response to the uniformly poor outcomes when patients undergo ReTx for acute events like primary graft failure. In this context, the median survival of patients undergoing cardiac transplantation has increased from 8.5 years in the era of 1982–1991 to almost 12 years for patients transplanted between 2002 and 2008. Median survival is even longer in young patients, with a median sur-vival of 12.6 years in patients undergoing initial transplant between age 18 and 39, compared to 9.1 years in patients aged 60–69. Patients under age 40 comprise 17% of the adult heart transplant population, but also represent the population most likely to require to eventually require ReTx. There is no reason to believe that there will not be an ongoing trend towards improved survival, potentially increasing the number of patients considered for ReTx.

Most of the data regarding the epidemiology of ReTx is only reflective of patients who success-fully undergo ReTx. Therefore, in order to demonstrate the potential increase in candidates for ReTx, we have provided an estimate based on outcomes in current transplant recipients, shown in **Figure 1**. Currently 74% of patients are surviving at least 5 years after their initial transplant date [5]. We will assume that patients who die before this time are not candidates for ReTx given poor outcomes in patients undergoing ReTx for acute graft failure. The pro-portion of patients who are over age 60 at the time of initial cardiac transplant is 23.8% [5]. For the sake of a conservative estimate, we will assume that these patients are not candidates for ReTx due to advanced age. In patients who die more than 5 years after transplant, CAV accounts for 7–17% of deaths and graft dysfunction accounts for 22–40% of deaths [5]. If all patients under age 60 at initial transplant who eventually die from CAV or graft dysfunction are assessed for ReTx, then 17% of all transplant patients could potentially be ReTx eligible. There are several assumptions built into this estimate. Many patients who are potential ReTx candidates due to CAV will not be eligible due to sudden death [8], or co-morbidities that preclude ReTx. However, if even half of the patients we estimated undergo ReTx this would essentially triple the current rate of ReTx.

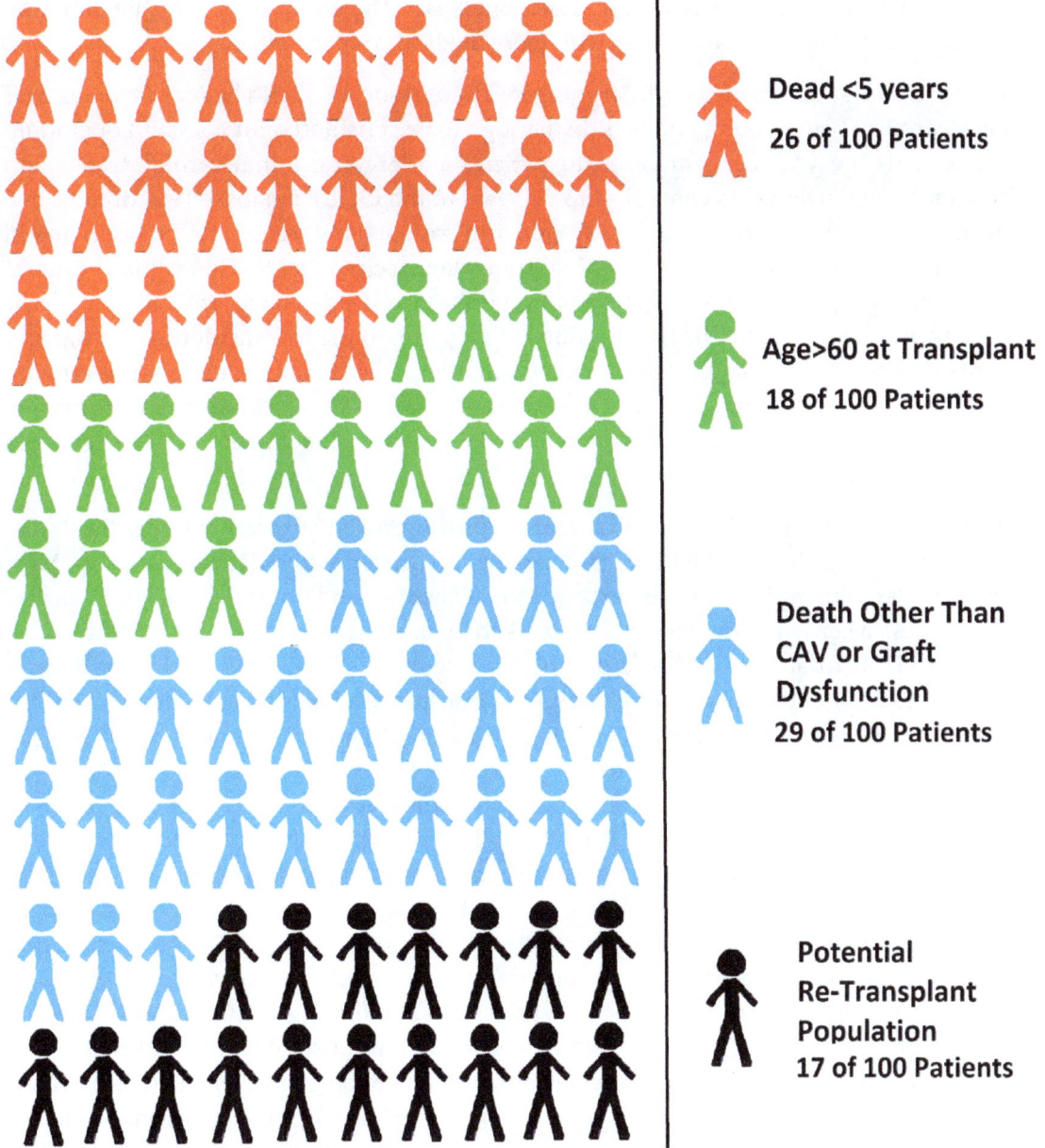

Figure 1. Estimate of the number of patients who may be candidates for cardiac ReTx. Estimates are based on ISHLT registry data [5, 9].

3. Characteristics of cardiac re-transplant recipients

Patients who undergo ReTx have characteristics distinct from those undergoing initial transplant. Some of these characteristics are related to procedures and immunosuppression required for the initial cardiac transplant. Meanwhile, other characteristics are related to surviving long enough to be considered for ReTx. However, as noted previously, this data only reflects patients who have successfully undergone ReTx. The group of patients who may be considered candidates are likely older with more medical co-morbidities.

Many characteristics of patients undergoing ReTx are associated with better outcomes, and generally reflect being young and healthy enough to be considered for a second operation. ReTx patients are younger compared to patients undergoing initial cardiac transplant, with a mean age of 46 years compared to 54 years in the ISHLT database [9]. Amiodarone exposure at any time point is also less frequent in patients undergoing ReTx, occurring in 10% of patients compared to 32% of initial transplant recipients [9]. This is interesting in light of emerging evidence suggesting amiodarone use is associated with higher 1-year mortality after transplant [10]. This finding is likely due to the low incidence of atrial and ventricular arrhythmias in the transplant population [11]. Finally, patients undergoing ReTx have lower pulmonary vascular resistance compared to other indications for transplant [5]. Overall these characteristics reflect the selection bias inherent in selection of ReTx candidates.

In ReTx populations, the characteristics that predict improved survival after cardiac transplant are more than outweighed by characteristics associated with adverse outcomes. Most patients undergoing ReTx have been exposed to calcineurin inhibitors after the initial cardiac transplant. As a consequence, they are more likely to have hypertension and renal dysfunction. In the ISHLT database 15.6% of patients undergoing ReTx had received prior dialysis compared to 3.9% in patients undergoing initial transplant [9]. Baseline creatinine was also higher in the ReTx group, 1.6 mg/dl compared to 1.2 mg/dL in initial transplant patients [9]. Hypertension is present in 57% of ReTx compared to 46% of initial transplant patients [9]. Additionally, ReTx patients have been exposed to a previous allograft and blood products during the initial cardiac transplant. Due to previous exposures, patients undergoing ReTx are more likely to be sensitized or highly sensitized. Almost 10% of patients undergoing ReTx have a Panel of Reactive Antibodies (PRA) greater than 80% compared to 2% of the primary transplant group [9]. Conversely, less than 50% of ReTx patients have a PRA of 0 compared to 65% of initial transplant patients [9]. High degrees of sensitization may complicate ReTx, requiring desensitization treatments prior to transplant or more aggressive induction therapy after transplant. All patients undergoing ReTx have had a prior sternotomy, which increases operative mortality as well as increasing cardiopulmonary bypass time, which increases morbidity and 90 day mortality associated with the operation [12, 13]. Finally, patients undergoing ReTx are more likely to be hospitalized at time of transplant, with 52% of ReTx patients admitted at the time of transplant compared to 44% of initial transplant patients [9]. This may reflect a trigger point for considering ReTx. These factors highlight the high risk nature of the ReTx population.

The characteristics outlined above reflect the population of patients who successfully undergo ReTx. The broader population of patients who may have been considered candidates for ReTx includes patients who may be too old, have co-morbidities that result in prohibitive risk, or are too highly sensitized to be successfully matched for ReTx. This suggests that, overall, the population considered for ReTx will be at significantly higher risk for peri-operative, short-term, and long-term complications after transplantation.

4. Patient outcomes following cardiac re-transplantation

There have been several attempts to characterize outcomes after ReTx. These studies span several eras of transplant management and reflect temoporal changes in patient selection criteria. What follows is not a comprehensive review of the available evidence, but a selected group of studies to highlight important concepts in the outcomes after ReTx.

4.1. Single-center studies

There have been several single-center studies outlining outcomes following ReTx, outlined in **Table 1**. Stanford reported a cohort of 66 patients who underwent ReTx before 1994 [14]. They found decreased one-year survival compared to primary heart transplant recipients (55 compared to 81%), with better survival in patients undergoing ReTx for CAV [14]. Schnetzler et al. investigated 24 patients who underwent ReTx before 1996 and found significantly reduced one-year survival for patient undergoing ReTx within a year (27.3%) compared to those undergoing ReTx after more than 1 year (61.5%) [15]. The patients transplanted within 1 year were exclusively patients with primary graft failure or intractable rejection [15]. A group from Columbia described a cohort of 43 patients undergoing ReTx before 1997 where 1-year and 5-year survival were decreased (66 vs. 76% and 51 vs. 60%) compared to initial transplant recipients [16]. They found that a shorter interval between ReTx and initial transplant as well as initial transplant for ischemic cardiomyopathy were associated with increased mortality compared to patients without those factors [16]. They

Author	Year	Center	Patients	Results
Smith	1995	Stanford	66 (26 acute, 40 chronic)	1-year survival 55% (vs 81%), 5-year survival 33% (vs 62%)
Schnetzler	1998	Paris	24 (11 acute, 13 chronic)	1-year survival 45.5% (vs. 71.6%), 5-year survival 31.2% (vs. 63.4%)
John	1999	Columbia	43 (13 within 2 years, 30 after 2 years)	1-year survival 66% (vs 76%), 5-year survival 51% (vs. 60%).
Schlechta	2001	Vienna	31 (16 acute, 15 chronic)	1-year survival 48.2% (vs. 80.2%), 5-year survival 36.8% (vs. 66.6%)
Topkara	2005	Columbia	41 patients	1-year survival 72.2% (vs. 85.5%), 5-year survival 47.5 (vs. 72.9%)
Alturi	2008	Pennsylvania	15 patients (11 chronic, 4 acute)	1-year survival 86.6% (vs 90.9%), 5-year survival 71.4% (vs. 79.1%)
Goerler	2008	Hannover	41 (18 acute, 23 chronic)	1-year survival 64% (vs. 83%), 5-year survival 47% (vs 72%)
Saito	2013	London, Ontario	22 (12 acute, 10 chronic)	Conditional 1-year survival 93.3% (vs. 93.0%) if surviving 30 days

Table 1. Single-center studies of re-transplant survival.

hypothesized that patients with ischemic cardiomyopathy may have atherosclerotic disease in other vascular beds leading to worse outcomes [16]. They also found improved survival in their population after excluding patients with acute graft failure and significant renal dysfunction [16]. A cohort of patients undergoing ReTx between 1984 and 1999 from Vienna had one-year survival as low as 48.2% in a cohort that was almost evenly split between acute and chronic indications for ReTx [17]. The authors suggested younger age, lack of peripheral vascular disease, and ability to actively rehabilitate after the primary transplant as criteria for ReTx candidacy [17]. These early studies were essential to identify the factors that influence survival, leading to better patient outcomes.

More contemporary cohorts have shown some improvement in ReTx outcomes through more rigorous patient selection. A single-center study from Germany reported a cohort of 41 patients who underwent ReTx prior to July 2006 [18]. Of those patients 18 underwent ReTx for acute graft failure and 23 for chronic graft failure [18]. They found decreased 1-year (64 compared to 83%) and 5-year survival (47 compared to 72%) in patients undergoing ReTx compared to initial transplant [18]. This finding was driven by high 30-day mortality (34.1 vs. 9.5%) in patients undergoing ReTx [18]. In their cohort, patients with chronic graft failure had better survival than those with acute graft failure as an indication for ReTx [18]. In a smaller Canadian study including patients transplanted bettween 1981 and 2011, patients who were retransplanted more than 1 year after initial implant had similar survival as patients undergoing initial transplantation [19]. Columbia reported improved survival in patients transplanted between 1992 and 2002 after selecting groups of patients with mostly CAV as the indication for ReTx [20]. The University of Pennsylvania heart transplant program had a similar experience in patients undergoing ReTx between 1987 and 2007 [20, 21]. While survival following ReTx is still lower compared to initial transplant patients, further improvements in patient selection may continue to decrease this disparity.

4.2. Registry studies

Survival after cardiac retransplantation has also been assessed using registry data, outlined in **Table 2**. An analysis from the International Society of Heart and Lung Transplant (ISHLT) database identified a total of 514 patients undergoing ReTx between 1987 and 1998, of whom more than 50% underwent ReTx for CAV. [22]. In this population, one-year survival was only 65%, but was higher after excluding patients who underwent ReTx within 2 years of the initial transplant [22]. However, post-transplant survival remained inferior in the subset of patients undergoing ReTx for chronic graft failure compared to patients undergoing initial transplant [22]. Patients undergoing ReTx at a low-volume center, older recipient age, and requiring ICU care prior to ReTx were associated with increased mortality [22]. An analysis of 107 patients undergoing ReTx between 1990 and 1999 in the Cardiac Transplant Research Database reported 56% 1-year survival [23]. In this cohort, patients undergoing ReTx for acute graft failure had 1-year survival of 50%, and in patients with acute rejection 1-year survival was even lower at 32% [23]. However, they found that retransplantation for CAV was associated with better survival with improvements in survival over time [23]. In the most recent analysis of the ISHLT database, patients undergoing ReTx between 2006 and June 2013 had one-year survival of 70%, but patients undergoing ReTx for primary graft failure had a one-year survival

Author	Year	Registry	Patients	Results
Srivasta	2000	ISHLT	514 patients (155 acute, 359 chronic)	1-year survival 65%, 3-year survival 55%
Radovancevic	2002	CTRD	107 patients (49 acute, 58 chronic)	1-year survival 56%, 5-year survival 38%
Lund	2014	ISHLT	820 patients (77% chronic, 23% acute)	1-year survival 70%, 5-year survival 54%

Table 2. Registry studies of re-transplant survival.

of 46% [9]. By comparison, patients undergoing ReTx for CAV had a one-year survival of 74% [23]. These studies highlight the importance of considering the indication for ReTx, which is a consistent predictor of mortality after correcting for other patient factors.

4.3. Outcomes in the pediatric population

Survival after ReTx is also strongly influenced by the age of the recipient. Therefore, authors have suspected that survival in the pediatric population may be better compared to adult populations. Select studies are outlined in **Table 3**. Razzouk et al. reported a cohort of 12 pediatric patients undergoing ReTx between 1985 and 1997 [24]. They found similar 1-year survival in patients undergoing ReTx compared to patients undergoing initial cardiac transplant [24]. Dearani et al. reported an updated cohort from the same center including 22 patients who underwent ReTx before 1999 [25]. One-year and 3-year survival was numerically, but not statistically, superior compared to initial transplant patients, with 3-year survival of 81.9 compared to 77.3% [25]. A cohort of 26 pediatric ReTx patients from Denver had similar one-year survival of 83% [26]. Conway et al. identified patients who underwent initial cardiac transplantation before age 18 in the ISHLT database [7]. They identified 602 patients who underwent ReTx between 1988 and 2010 and found that early mortality was similar to patients undergoing initial cardiac transplant, with a hazard ratio of only 1.07 [7]. However, patients undergoing ReTx were more likely to develop CAV, late rejection, and late renal dysfunction [7]. An important consideration in this group is that pediatric patients who are listed on adult transplant waitlists will wait for a longer period of time and are more likely to die on the waitlist [27]. Given

Author	Year	Center/registry	Patients	Results
Razzouk	1998	Loma Linda	12 patients	1-year survival 84.3 (vs. 83.3%), 4-year survival 74.4 (vs 83.3%)
Dearani	2001	Loma Linda	22 (16 chronic, 6 acute)	1-year survival 81.9% (vs 84.1%), 3-year survival 81.9% (vs 77.3%)
Karamichalis	2011	Denver	26 (10 chronic, 16 acute)	1-year survival 83%, 5-year survival 67%
Conway	2014	ISHLT	602 (acute and chronic)	1-year survival 83%, 5-year survival 69%

Table 3. Pediatric studies of re-transplant survival.

the improved proportional survival of pediatric ReTx patients compared to adult cohorts, it is likely that outcomes will also be acceptable in the younger adult population.

5. Patient selection for cardiac re-transplantation

The Consensus Conference on Retransplantation was sponsored by the American Society of Transplantation, the American Society of Transplant Surgeons, and the National Institute of Allergy and Infectious Diseases and was held in Atlanta in 2006 and outlined several important considerations for ReTx candidacy [6]. The working group concluded that patients undergoing ReTx should have either chronic graft failure in the absence of active rejection, or severe CAV not amenable to medical or surgical therapy. Additionally they suggested that patients with CAV should have either symptoms attributable to CAV or moderate to severe left ventricular dysfunction. Additionally, they proposed that patients with graft failure due to ongoing acute rejection, especially less than 6 months post-transplant, be ineligible for ReTx. In addition to considerations regarding the indication for ReTx, there are several other patient factors that warrant discussion given their strong associations with survival following ReTx.

Patient selection is a key component for improving short and long-term survival following ReTx. A summary of factors known to be associated with patient outcomes is presented in **Table 4**. Long-term survival is strongly driven by age at time of ReTx, as evidenced by relatively good outcomes seen in pediatric populations. Given the impact of age on survival, some groups have questioned the efficacy of ReTx in patients over the age of 60 years [6]. Patients undergoing ReTx have longer exposure to immunosuppression which may explain a possible increase in the risk of infections and malignancies; [28] therefore, careful attention should be given to excluding infection or occult malignancy when assessing ReTx candidacy. Poor renal function is also more common in ReTx patients and is associated with increased mortality. In a cohort of ReTx patients from Stanford, patients with creatinine >2.0 mg/dL had worse short-term outcomes, while patients undergoing simultaneous heart and kidney transplant had improved survival [14]. Similarly, patients on hemodialysis undergoing initial cardiac transplant in the UNOS database had better survival when undergoing simultaneous

Associated with worse patient outcomes	Associated with improved patient outcomes
Shorter interval between initial transplant and ReTx (<6 months)	Younger age
Primary/acute graft failure	Lack of peripheral vascular disease
Ischemic cardiomyopathy	CAV/Chronic graft failure
Renal dysfunction (Creatinine >2.0 mg/dL)	
Multiple previous sternotomies	
Requiring ICU care pre-operatively	

Table 4. Summary of predictors associated with patient outcomes.

heart-kidney transplant compared heart transplant alone [29]. Therefore, poor renal function should be considered a relative contraindication to ReTx unless the patient is a candidate for simultaneous heart-kidney transplant.

The number of previous sternotomies should also be considered when deciding if a patient is a candidate for ReTx. Multiple previous sternotomies from prior palliative congenital procedures or coronary artery bypass grafting adds to the burden of scar tissue, in addition to potentially complicated anastamotic sites from the initial transplant. Some authors have argued that this contributes to the high rates of multi-system organ failure in patients after ReTx, as well as high rates of early mortality [18, 28]. These findings are attributed to an increased incidence of mediastinitis, intrathoracic bleeding requiring reintervention, and primary graft failure [30]. These findings have also been seen in pediatric ReTx, many of which have had previous palliative procedures [26]. Lastly, patients admitted to ICU prior to ReTx, and particularly those requiring mechanical circulatory support, have worse outcomes [31]. In these patients it is important to not only ensure that organ dysfunction is reversible, but also that the patient will be capable of undergoing rehabilitation if the operation is successful. Consideration of these factors may help identify patients with the greatest potential benefit from ReTx.

Patients undergoing ReTx are more highly sensitized than patients undergoing initial cardiac transplant [5]. Higher sensitization increases the risk of CAV, acute rejection and post-transplant mortality [32, 33]. Therefore, it may be necessary to consider options to desensitize patients prior to ReTx in order to improve the chance of successful graft matching as well as improving outcomes following ReTx.

6. Management of patients following re-transplantation

Many studies have highlighted the high early mortality seen after ReTx and patient factors that might be driving this observation. This may reflect the increased complexity of the surgical operation as well as medical frailty in patients undergoing ReTx, but highlights the importance of careful early management. As mentioned previously, the most important aspect of patient management is careful selection of patients who are likely to benefit from ReTx. However, once an appropriate patient has been selected, it is important to optimize the perioperative care in order to attain the best possible outcomes.

From a surgical perspective, it is important to identify the surgical technique used in the initial transplant. It may be especially pertinent to determine if the patient underwent bicaval or bi-atrial anastomosis as well as the level of anastomosis of the pulmonary artery and aorta. Dedicated thoracic imaging, either computed tomographic or magnetic resonance, may help identify anastomotic sites and areas with significant fibrotic tissue. It is not clear if it is necessary to completely excise all of the tissue from the initial cardiac transplant and no guidelines exist to advise clinical practice. Theoretically, it may help to reduce the potential for immunogenicity in those patients; however, this benefit needs to be weighed against increasing the complexity of the operation, which could potentially prolong bypass time and increase peri-operative complications. Finally, careful attention to hemostasis is important as always, but may be particularly important in ReTx patients in whom peri-operative bleeding is more frequent.

There are no clear guidelines on the post-operative care for patients undergoing ReTx. Theoretically, it may not be necessary to add induction therapy if patients have been maintained on high doses of immunosuppression, since their immune response is already significantly blunted. This is not the case for patients undergoing ReTx for refractory rejection or patients who are highly sensitized. However, most transplant centers have used similar induction and immunosuppressive regimens for their primary transplant and ReTx patients. Following induction, it may be reasonable to de-escalate immunosuppression more quickly than would be typical after initial transplantation in order to reduce the long-term risks associated with malignancy and infection.

7. Alternative therapies

Unfortunately, there are no established alternatives to ReTx for patients who have developed late complications of cardiac transplantation. There are no effective strategies for managing end-stage CAV and mortality rates are very high. Similarly, there are no established medical therapies for patients who have developed late graft dysfunction. Columbia has reported the use of mechanical circulatory support as a bridge to re-transplantation [34]. However, given the prevalence of restrictive filling dynamics and right ventricular dysfunction, long-term mechanical support is unlikely to be successful in many patients. Therefore, there are no clearly viable alternatives to ReTx and the default therapy has been, and will continue to be, palliative care. Therefore, it is important to review end-of-life planning and consider palliative care consultation in patients who develop long-term complications.

8. Ethical considerations in re-transplantation

A complete discussion of the ethical considerations of ReTx beyond the scope of this chapter and readers would be well-served to read dedicated manuscripts [18, 35–37]. Donor hearts are a limited resource and need to be valued appropriately. The number of patients listed for cardiac transplantation greatly outstrips this supply and will continue to do so until we use a much larger proportion of potential donor hearts, an alternate source of grafts is established, or fewer patients require cardiac transplantation. None of these events are likely to occur in the near future. Given the ongoing scarcity of donor hearts, it is important to offer organs to those patients who would derive the most benefit. This is a strong argument against ReTx for acute indications, where outcomes are consistently poor. ReTx for CAV or chronic graft dysfunction is also associated with worse survival compared to initial transplantation, but it is not clear if this is a sufficient reason to exclude all ReTx. Finally, there has been concern regarding the possible injustice inherent in ReTx. Many patients will not survive to receive a single heart transplant and it may not seem equitable for a single patient to receive two, or even three organs when there are patients who die before receiving their first. This debate will continue, but if clinical outcomes continue to improve in ReTx populations, there may be a shift towards broader acceptance of this procedure.

9. Conclusions

ReTx represents a small proportion of heart transplant procedures today; however, survival following cardiac transplantation has improved dramatically and more patients are surviving until they develop late complications such as CAV or graft failure. ReTx is the only therapy that offers meaningful improvement in survival to these patients. Survival after ReTx seems to be reduced, but may be acceptable in appropriately chosen patients. Tailored surgical and post-operative care is critical to improving patient outcomes in those accepted for ReTx.

Conflict of interest

The authors have no relevant conflicts of interest to declare.

Author details

Robert JH Miller* and Kiran Khush

*Address all correspondence to: rjhmille@stanford.edu

Department of Medicine, Stanford University, Division of Cardiovascular Medicine, Palo Alto, California, United States

References

[1] Lund LH, Khush KK, Cherikh WS, et al. The registry of the International Society for Heart and Lung Transplantation: Thirty-fourth adult heart transplantation Report-2017; focus theme: Allograft ischemic time. The Journal of Heart and Lung Transplantation. 2017;**36**:1037-1046

[2] Mehra MR. Contemporary concepts in prevention and treatment of cardiac allograft vasculopathy. American Journal of Transplantation. 2006;**6**:1248-1256

[3] Magee JC, Barr ML, Basadonna GP, et al. Repeat organ transplantation in the United States, 1996-2005. American Journal of Transplantation. 2007;**7**:1424-1433

[4] Goldraich LA, Stehlik J, Kucheryavaya AY, Edwards LB, Ross HJ. Retransplant and medical therapy for cardiac allograft vasculopathy: International Society for Heart and Lung Transplantation registry analysis. American Journal of Transplantation. 2016;**16**:301-309

[5] Lund LH, Edwards LB, Dipchand AI, et al. The registry of the International Society for Heart and Lung Transplantation: Thirty-third adult heart transplantation report-2016; Focus theme: Primary diagnostic indications for transplant. The Journal of Heart and Lung Transplantation. 2016;**35**:1158-1169

[6] Johnson MR, Aaronson KD, Canter CE, et al. Heart retransplantation. American Journal of Transplantation. 2007;**7**:2075-2081

[7] Conway J, Manlhiot C, Kirk R, Edwards LB, McCrindle BW, Dipchand AI. Mortality and morbidity after retransplantation after primary heart transplant in childhood: An analysis from the registry of the International Society for Heart and Lung Transplantation. The Journal of Heart and Lung Transplantation. 2014;**33**:241-251

[8] Baris N, Sipahi I, Kapadia SR, et al. Coronary angiography for follow-up of heart transplant recipients: Insights from TIMI frame count and TIMI myocardial perfusion grade. The Journal of Heart and Lung Transplantation. 2007;**26**:593-597

[9] Lund LH, Edwards LB, Kucheryavaya AY, et al. The registry of the International Society for Heart and Lung Transplantation: Thirty-first official adult heart transplant report--2014; focus theme: Retransplantation. The Journal of Heart and Lung Transplantation. 2014; **33**:996-1008

[10] Cooper LB, Mentz RJ, Edwards LB, et al. Amiodarone use in patients listed for heart transplant is associated with increased 1-year post-transplant mortality. The Journal of Heart and Lung Transplantation. 2017;**36**:202-210

[11] Chang HY, Lo LW, Feng AN, et al. Long-term follow-up of arrhythmia characteristics and clinical outcomes in heart transplant patients. Transplantation Proceedings. 2013; **45**:369-375

[12] Ott GY, Norman DJ, Hosenpud JD, Hershberger RE, Ratkovec RM, Cobanoglu A. Heart transplantation in patients with previous cardiac operations. The Journal of Thoracic and Cardiovascular Surgery. 1994;**107**:203-209

[13] George TJ, Beaty CA, Ewald GA, et al. Reoperative sternotomy is associated with increased mortality after heart transplantation. The Annals of Thoracic Surgery. 2012;**94**: 2025-2032

[14] Smith JA, Ribakove GH, Hunt SA, et al. Heart retransplantation: The 25-year experience at a single institution. The Journal of Heart and Lung Transplantation. 1995;**14**:832-839

[15] Schnetzler BMD, Pavie AMD, Dorent RMD, et al. Heart retransplantation: A 23-year single-center clinical experience. The Annals of Thoracic Surgery. 1998;**65**:978-983

[16] John R, Chen JM, Weinberg A, et al. Long-term survival after cardiac retransplantation: A twenty-year single-center experience. The Journal of Thoracic and Cardiovascular Surgery. 1999;**117**:543-555

[17] Schlechta B, Kocher AA, Ehrlich M, et al. Heart retransplantation: Institutional results of a series of 31 cases. Transplantation Proceedings. 2001;**33**:2759-2761

[18] Goerler H, Simon A, Gohrbandt B, et al. Cardiac retransplantation: Is it justified in times of critical donor organ shortage? Long-term single-center experience. European Journal of Cardio-Thoracic Surgery. 2008;**34**:1185-1190

[19] Saito A, Novick RJ, Kiaii B, et al. Early and late outcomes after cardiac retransplantation. Canadian Journal of Surgery. 2013;**56**:21-26

[20] Topkara VK, Dang NC, John R, et al. A decade experience of cardiac retransplantation in adult recipients. The Journal of heart and lung transplantation : the official publication of the International Society for Heart Transplantation. 2005;**24**:1745-1750

[21] Atluri P, Hiesinger W, Gorman RC, et al. Cardiac retransplantation is an efficacious therapy for primary cardiac allograft failure. Journal of Cardiothoracic Surgery. 2008;**3**:26-26

[22] Srivastava R, Keck BM, Bennett LE, Hosenpud JD. The results of cardiac retransplantation: An analysis of the Joint International Society for Heart and Lung Transplantation/ United Network for Organ Sharing Thoracic Registry. Transplantation. 2000;**70**:606-612

[23] Radovancevic B, McGiffin DC, Kobashigawa JA, et al. Retransplantation in 7,290 primary transplant patients: A 10-year multi-institutional study. The Journal of Heart and Lung Transplantation. 2003;**22**:862-868

[24] Razzouk AJ, Chinnock RE, Dearani JA, Gundry SR, Bailey LL. Cardiac retransplantation for graft vasculopathy in children: Should we continue to do it? Archives of Surgery. 1998;**133**:881-885

[25] Dearani JA, Razzouk AJ, Gundry SR, et al. Pediatric cardiac retransplantation: Intermediate-term results. The Annals of Thoracic Surgery. 2001;**71**:66-70

[26] Karamichalis JM, Miyamoto SD, Campbell DN, et al. Pediatric cardiac retransplant: Differing patterns of primary graft failure by age at first transplant. The Journal of Thoracic and Cardiovascular Surgery. 2011;**141**:223-230

[27] Bock MJ, Nguyen K, Malerba S, et al. Pediatric cardiac retransplantation: Waitlist mortality stratified by age and era. The Journal of Heart and Lung Transplantation. 2015; **34**:530-537

[28] Tsao L, Uriel N, Leitz K, Naka Y, Mancini D. Higher rate of comorbidities after cardiac Retransplantation contributes to decreased survival. The Journal of Heart and Lung Transplantation. 2009;**28**:1072-1074

[29] Gill J, Shah T, Hristea I, et al. Outcomes of simultaneous heart-kidney transplant in the US: A retrospective analysis using OPTN/UNOS data. American Journal of Transplantation. 2009;**9**:844-852

[30] Hosenpud JD, Novick RJ, Bennett LE, Keck BM, Fiol B, Daily OP. The registry of the International Society for Heart and Lung Transplantation: Thirteenth official report—1996. The Journal of Heart and Lung Transplantation. 1996;**15**:655-674

[31] Belli E, Leoni Moreno JC, Hosenpud J, Rawal B, Landolfo K. Preoperative risk factors predict survival following cardiac retransplantation: Analysis of the United Network for Organ Sharing database. The Journal of Thoracic and Cardiovascular Surgery. 2014; **147**:1972-1977

[32] Kaczmarek I, Deutsch MA, Kauke T, et al. Donor-specific HLA alloantibodies: Long-term impact on cardiac allograft vasculopathy and mortality after heart transplant. Experimental and Clinical Transplantation. 2008;6:229-235

[33] Nwakanma LU, Williams JA, Weiss ES, Russell SD, Baumgartner WA, Conte JV. Influence of pretransplant panel-reactive antibody on outcomes in 8,160 heart transplant recipients in recent era. The Annals of Thoracic Surgery. 2007;84:1556-1563

[34] Clerkin KJ, Thomas SS, Haythe J, et al. Mechanical circulatory support as a bridge to cardiac retransplantation: A single center experience. The Journal of Heart and Lung Transplantation: The Official Publication of the International Society for Heart Transplantation. 2015;34:161-166

[35] Haddad H. Cardiac retransplantation: An ethical dilemma. Current Opinion in Cardiology. 2006;21:118-119

[36] Luquire R, Houston S. Ethical concerns regarding cardiac retransplantation. Nursing Economics. 1992;10:413-417

[37] Collins EG, Mozdzierz GJ. Cardiac retransplantation: Determining limits. Heart & Lung: The Journal of Critical Care. 1993;22:206-212

6

Humoral Rejection in Cardiac Transplantation: Management of Antibody-Mediated Rejection

Umit Kervan, Dogan Emre Sert and Nesrin Turan

Abstract

After a successful heart transplantation, fundamental keys to achieve good results in the long term are to establish immunosuppressive therapy in the postoperative period in an appropriate manner and to ensure continuity of follow-ups. Despite the fact that these stages are maintained perfectly, patients may face one or more rejection episodes. T-cell-mediated acute cellular rejection of the cardiac allograft has well-established treatment algorithms, whereas antibody-mediated rejection (AMR) is challenging to diagnose, and its treatment varies between centers. Investigators reported that AMR is among the most important factors to improving long-term outcomes. Improved understanding of the roles of acute and chronic AMR has evolved in recent years following a major progress in the technical ability to detect and quantify recipient antihuman leukocyte antigen (HLA) antibody production. Recently, a study of the immunobiology of B cells and plasma cells that pertains to allograft rejection and tolerance has emerged. There are some questions regarding the classification of AMR, the diagnostic approaches, and the treatment strategies for managing. In this chapter, we are discuss the effector mechanisms that are used by antibodies to eliminate antigens and clinical experience about AMR and its treatment with a discussion about the latest articles.

Keywords: heart transplantation, rejection, humoral, plasmapheresis, rituximab

1. Introduction

Orthotopic heart transplantation (OHT) is still the gold standard of treatment among end-stage heart failure. Worldwide, about 3500 heart transplantations are performed annually [1]. However, shortage of donors and allograft dysfunction are the most common problems cardiac surgeons have to cope with. Rejection is the most common reason for allograft dysfunction and is responsible for 25% of postoperative deaths [2]. Episodes of rejection may emerge at any time after transplantation as acute or chronic cellular rejection (CR), humoral rejection (=antibody-mediated = vascular rejection (AMR)), or mixed rejection. Despite AMR that is known to be rare, it is potentially lethal due to the capillary vasculopathy caused by neutrophil and macrophage infiltration in endothelial cells [3, 4]. Today, treatment of rejection episodes is directed mostly to cellular response. Each center sets the treatment in the light of their experience. In this chapter, we will discuss the effector mechanisms that are used by antibodies to eliminate antigens and clinical experience about AMR and its treatment with discussing the latest articles.

2. Overview of humoral immunity

Antibodies are accumulated by the immune system to identify and neutralize foreign objects. They were the first specific product of the adaptive immune response to be identified and are found in the plasma, in the blood, and in extracellular fluids. Immunity mediated by antibodies is known as humoral immunity because of body fluids that were once known as humors [4]. The humoral immune response begins with the recognition of antigens by native B cells. These cells then undergo a process of clonal expansion and differentiation. In this way, the B cell matures into antibody-secreting plasma cells, which secrete antibodies. The activation of B cells and their differentiation into antibody-secreting plasma cells is triggered by antigen and usually requires helper T cells. The term "helper T cell" is often used to mean a cell from the TH2 class of CD4 T cells, but a subset of TH1 cells can also help in B-cell activation [5]. B cells can receive help from helper T cells when antigen bound by surface immunoglobulin is internalized and returned to the cell surface as peptides bound to major histocompatibility complex (MHC) class II molecules. MHC then delivers activating signals to the B cell. Thus, protein antigens binding to B cells both provide a specific signal to the B cell by cross-linking its antigen receptors and allow the B cell to attract antigen-specific T-cell help. These antigens are unable to induce antibody responses in animals or humans who lack T cells, and they are therefore known as thymus-dependent antigens [5]. The first signal required for B-cell activation is delivered through its antigen receptor. For thymus-dependent antigens, the second signal is delivered by a helper T cell that recognizes degraded fragments of the antigen as peptides bound to MHC class II molecules on the B-cell surface; the interaction between CD40 ligand on the T cell and CD40 on the B cell contributes an essential part of this second signal [5]. For thymus-independent antigens, the second signal can be delivered by the antigen itself or by non-thymus-derived accessory cells. The B-cell co-receptor complex of CD19:CD21:CD81 can greatly enhance B-cell responsiveness to antigen. CD21 (=complement receptor 2) is a receptor for the complement fragment C3d. Whether binding of CD21 enhances B-cell responsiveness by increasing B-cell signaling, by inducing co-stimulatory molecules on the B cell, or by increasing the receptor-mediated uptake of antigen is not yet known [5]. Antibodies are the effector products of humoral immunity. Finally, as this response declines, a pool of memory cells remains behind. If the body is reexposed to the antigen, these memory cells will recognize the antigen and respond much more quickly and effectively [6]. There are two purposes of antibodies. The first purpose is to neutralize the target threat, and the second purpose is to recruit other cells or proteins to an antigen so that those cells or proteins can eliminate the antigen [6]. AMR develops when recipient antibody is directed against donor human leukocyte antigens (HLA) on the endothelial layer of the allograft. Antibodies induce fixation and activation of the complement cascade, resulting in tissue injury. Complement and immunoglobulin are deposited within the allograft microvasculature, which results in an inflammatory process that is characterized by endothelial cell activation, upregulation of cytokines, infiltration of macrophages, increased vascular permeability, and microvascular thrombosis. This process ultimately manifests as allograft dysfunction [6].

3. Humoral rejection (=antibody-mediated = vascular rejection (AMR))

AMR is mediated by donor-specific antibodies and is histologically defined by linear deposits of immunoglobulin (Ig) and complement in the myocardial capillaries [7]. Herskowitz et al. [8] described AMR for the first time in 1987 as an arteriolar vasculitis with poor outcome. Hammond et al. [9] firstly demonstrated that vascular rejection is associated with deposits of antibodies and complement activation. AMR incidence is reported between 8 and 15% [10–12], and it has been reported concurrent with CR in up to 24% of cases. Approximately 50% of heart transplant recipients who develop rejection >7 years after transplantation have evidence of AMR [12]. AMR was described as an acute phenomenon seen in weeks to months just after OHT. However, in recent years, studies have been reported that it also occurs in the longer term [9, 13, 14]. Rejection can be hyperacute (occurring within minutes after the vascular anastomosis (0–7 days)) in patients who are sensitized to donor HLA antigens and acute (occurring days to weeks after transplantation) because of the development of de novo donor-specific antibody (DSA) and preexisting DSA. Early AMR tends to be associated with a higher prevalence of allograft dysfunction and hemodynamic compromise. Late (occurring 3 months after transplantation) or chronic rejection most likely because of heightened recognition (occurring months to years after transplantation) [15]. Risk factors include young age, female gender, high levels of pretransplant panel-reactive antibodies (PRAs), positive donor-specific crossmatch, cytomegalovirus infection, prior OKT3 use, and artificial heart devices [10, 13]. Olsen et al. [16] stated that 23% of patients had AMR episodes for the second time resulting in graft loss in two-thirds due to the continuous complement activation and production of donor-reactive antibodies that cause graft dysfunction by sensitized memory B cells. As the definition of AMR has evolved and more sensitive diagnostic modalities have become available, there is increasing evidence that AMR is a spectrum of immunologic injury that ranges from subclinical, histological, immunologic, and/or serological findings without graft dysfunction (i.e., subclinical AMR) to overt AMR with hemodynamic compromise.

3.1. Diagnosis

The first description of humoral rejection was included in the 1990 International Society of Heart and Lung Transplantation (ISHLT) criteria defined as positive immunofluorescence, vasculitis, or severe edema in the absence of cellular infiltrate [14, 17]. The classification AMR 0 was assigned in the absence of histological or immunopathologic features. Confirmation of

AMR or AMR 1 was defined as histological evidence with identification of antibodies (CD68, CD31, C4d) and serum presence of DSA [14]. ISHLT Immunopathology Task Force provided an expanded description of the histological evidence of acute capillary injury, the minimum requirement for immunopathologic evidence of antibody-mediated injury, and an improved definition of serological evidence of circulating antibodies in 2006 [18]. The persistent variations in the diagnosis and treatment of AMR were addressed in the Heart Session of the Tenth Banff Conference on Allograft Pathology (2009) and the ISHLT Consensus Conference on AMR (2010) conferences. The most important issues included the need for a clinical definition of AMR, the significance of asymptomatic patient without cardiac dysfunction biopsy-proven AMR, and the recognition that AMR may be caused by DSA as well as antibodies to non-HLA antigens. Although AMR would be a pathological diagnosis, it was strongly recommended that at the time of suspected AMR, blood can be drawn at biopsy and tested for the presence of donor-specific anti-HLA class I and class II antibodies [14]. On the basis of the initial Banff criteria, a definitive diagnosis of AMR required morphologic evidence (primarily microvascular inflammation), immunohistological (C4d staining), and serologic criteria (presence of circulating DSA). These criteria were modified to address the current evidence of the existence of C4d-negative AMR and lesions of intimal arteritis secondary to the action of the antibodies at the Banff Consensus in 2013 [19]. The myocardial capillaries, arterioles, and venules are readily sampled at biopsy. The vascular endothelium is the point of the first contact for anti-donor antibody in the allograft and the primary locus of activity in AMR. The appearance of vasculitis or leukocytes infiltrating through the endothelium into the vessel wall demonstrates active humoral immunity with antibody-dependent cytotoxicity, cytokine, and circulating monocyte recruitment [20, 21]. Mechanisms of immune complex-mediated neutrophil recruitment and tissue injury. Antibodies induce fixation and activation of the complement cascade, resulting in tissue injury. Complement activation, a key contributor to the pathogenesis of AMR, results in activation of the innate and adaptive immune responses. Complement and immunoglobulin are deposited within the allograft microvasculature, which results in an inflammatory process that is characterized by endothelial cell activation, upregulation of cytokines, infiltration of macrophages, increased vascular permeability, and microvascular thrombosis. Interstitial edema and hemorrhage are also seen. Capillary changes indicative of AMR include endothelial cell swelling and intravascular macrophage accumulation coincident with pericapillary neutrophils. The role of immunoglobulins, complement activation, and coagulation cascade in AMR is under constant study as diagnostic methods increase in sensitivity and specificity [14, 22]. It has been suggested that AMR is a clinical pathological continuum that begins with a latent humoral response of circulating antibodies and then progresses through a silent phase of circulating antibodies with C4d deposition without clinical or histological alterations, to a subclinical stage, to symptomatic AMR [14]. Mauiyyedi et al. described the correlation between DSAs and diffuse C4d deposition (>50%) as diagnostic markers for AMR [23]. C4d deposition may be earlier than 3 months, as may be after 160 months [7, 10, 24]. The complement components C3 and C1q have been demonstrated in kidney AMR; however, their detection is limited by a short half-life in vivo and consequently a short window of detection during a rejection episode [25]. The protein C4d is a complement split product that binds covalently to the endothelium at the site of complement activation and persists longer than C3 or C1q [14]. C4d and C3d detection predicts graft dysfunction and mortality better than C4d alone [14, 26]. Haas et al. reported that biopsies positive for C4d (C4d+) and C3d (C3d+) are strongly associated with DSA and allograft dysfunction, while cases with episodes that are only positive for C4d are mostly subclinical [19]. Berry et al. published working formulation by pathologists to diagnose "pathological AMR (pAMR)" without the requirement of clinical dysfunction or positive DSA (**Table 1**) [27, 28]. CD59 and CD55 (decay-accelerating factors) are used in conjunction with C4d and C3d to indicate aborted complement activation. Lengthy incubation times and a granular staining pattern render these assays impractical for clinical use [26]. The macrophage antigen CD68 allows identification of subtle accumulations of macrophages within vessels, which helps to differentiate intravascular/perivascular macrophages from lymphocytes, thereby excluding ACR. Because interstitial macrophages are commonly found in allograft myocardium in a variety of settings, including AMR, ACR, and ischemic injury, investigators agree that only macrophages within capillaries and small venules are to be considered [29]. The term "intravascular macrophage" was replaced by "activated mononuclear cells" because it was clear that without immunostaining with CD68, intravascular T lymphocytes and activated endothelial cells could be misinterpreted as macrophages at the 2012 ISHLT workshop [28]. Endothelial cell markers CD34 and CD31 can be used to ascertain the intravascular location of macrophages/mononuclear cells [30]. Immunopathologic features of AMR were summarized in **Table 2**. Using criteria that included prominent endothelial cell swelling and/or vasculitis and the vascular deposition of immunoglobulin and complement, it was first defined by Hammond and co-workers [9]. The clinic spectrum of AMR ranges from latent AMR to silent AMR, to subclinical AMR, and to clinical AMR. Pathologic evidence of AMR appears in silent AMR as C4d deposition in capillaries of an otherwise normal myocardium and progresses to subclinical AMR showing myocardial alterations in the setting of C4d deposition but the absence of organ dysfunction. The onset of allograft dysfunction is the hallmark of clinical AMR [28, 31].

3.1.1. Surveillance and frequency of immunopathologic assessment

Kfoury et al. recommended that immunostaining for C4d be avoided in the first 2 weeks after transplant because a number of perioperative issues can confound staining and interpretation [32]. Center-specific approaches to the issue of surveillance vary widely, ranging from none to every biopsy. The other question is follow-up of positive immunostaining after therapy of AMR. The ISHLT pathology group recommended that subsequent biopsies should be studied

Category	Description
pAMR 0: negative for pathological AMR	Both histological and immunopathologic studies are negative
pAMR 1 (H+): histopathologic AMR alone	Histological findings positive and immunopathologic findings negative
pAMR1 (I+): immunopathologic AMR alone	Histological findings negative and immunopathologic findings positive
pAMR 2: pathological AMR	Both histological and immunopathologic findings are present
pAMR 3: severe pathological AMR	Severe AMR with histopathologic findings of interstitial hemorrhage, capillary fragmentation, mixed inflammatory infiltrates, endothelial cell pyknosis and/or karyorrhexis, and marked edema

AMR, antibody-mediated rejection; pAMR, pathological AMR (Source: [28]).

Table 1. The 2013 ISHLT working formulation for pathologic diagnosis of cardiac antibody-mediated rejection.

	Interpretation	AMR limitations
IgG/IgM	Immunoglobulin binding	+ Easily dissociated, short half-life, interobserver variability
C3, C1q	Complement activation	+ Short half-life
C3d/C4d	Complement activation	+ Combination more predictive of AMR than C4d alone, long half-life
HLA-DR	Endothelial integrity	+ Staining always present, but "frayed" pattern indicates capillary injury
Fibrin	Thrombotic environment	+ Interstitial extravasation suggests more severe AMR episode
CD55, CD59	Complement inhibitor	− Long incubation and granular staining pattern, difficult to be interpreted
CD31, CD34, CD68	Intravascular macrophages	+ CD68 confirms macrophage lineage of mononuclear cells, CD31 and CD34 are endothelial markers which differentiate macrophages from endothelial cells and delineate intravascular localization

AMR, antibody-mediated rejection; HLA, human leukocyte antigens (Source: [14]).

Table 2. Immunopathologic features of antibody-mediated rejection.

by immunostaining until a negative result is achieved in 2011. However, investigators reported that capillary staining of C3d cleared within 2 weeks to 1 month, while capillary staining of C4d cleared within 1–2 months [26].

3.2. Treatment

Investigators have since reported on its incidence, histopathological features, clinical outcome, and treatment. However, clinical series are few and sparse, and the incidence of HR and the method of choice for its management remain uncertain and may differ among different centers [33]. All transplantation centers often prefer pulse steroid as an initial therapy in combination with plasmapheresis. Otherwise, intravenous cyclophosphamide (0.5 to 1 gm/m², every 3 weeks for 4–6 months) may be added to treatment regimen according to the clinical experience and preferences. In case of recurrent AMR exacerbations, cyclophosphamide and IVIg (250 mg/kg/day, 4 days, 4–6 months repeated every 3 weeks) followed by plasmapheresis (5–6 sessions, 10–14 days) have been suggested. After 2002, rituximab (375 mg/m², once a week, four dose infusions) after plasmapheresis is added to treatment regimen [34].

Plasmapheresis is the cornerstone in the treatment of AMR. Exchange method and double-filtration technique are among the most used plasmapheresis methods. Both techniques are nonselective and eliminate immunoglobulins nonspecifically. Immunoadsorption plasmapheresis method using adsorbent membrane is more specific to the removal of antibodies; however, it is expensive. Each type of plasmapheresis involves risks such as hypovolemia and infection [4, 35, 36].

Plasmapheresis has been always reported in combination with other immunosuppressive agents; there is always a possibility of AMR recurrence as a monotherapy. In this context, other therapies are to be combined in order to prevent recurrence.

Another issue which is also controversial regarding plasmapheresis is about the number of sessions of plasmapheresis to be made and at what intervals. General practice is three to five sessions every other day. However, Crespo-Leiro et al. [33] reported that they use plasmapheresis every day until the recovery of the clinical status. The author who reported this period may extend to the nineteenth day. We perform plasmapheresis every other day for three sessions, and if there is no clinical improvement, we extend it up to five sessions in our general practice. Cytolytic therapy would be useful especially for those who need inotropics or mechanical circulatory support [13, 16]. Cytolytic therapy may indirectly suppress B lymphocyte activation, whereas antithymocyte globulin may directly suppress B-cell function [37, 38].

CD20 protein is a molecule present on the surface of B lymphocytes. Rituximab is a chimeric monoclonal antibody raised against the CD20 protein. Combination of rituximab with plasmapheresis, IVIg, or steroids was found to increase the success of treatment [39, 40]. Complement blockade would be an important strategy for prevention and treatment of AMR. Agents targeting C5 and C1 esterase have been evaluated in clinical trials. Eculizumab binds to complement protein C5 and inhibits complement. It prevents the breakdown of C5 and formation of MAC. Since eculizumab cannot decrease the levels of donor-specific antigen, antibody-lowering therapy should be added. Although early studies on the effects of eculizumab are promising, the use of eculizumab is limited due to the cost and lack of coverage by most insurers [41, 42]. Plasma-derived human C1-inhibitor (20UI/kg/twice weekly), an inhibitor which targets the classical complement pathway, was successfully administered for caAMR prevention in highly sensitized patients [43, 44]. Two C1-INH products that are approved for use by the FDA in the treatment of hereditary angioedema have been evaluated in small pilot studies for AMR: Berinert® (CSL Behring, Kankakee, IL, USA) and Cinryze® (Shire ViroPharma Inc., Lexington, MA, USA) [45, 46, 47]. A potential limitation of available therapies for AMR is the lack of direct effect on the major alloantibody-producing plasma cell. In recent years, studies regarding bortezomib, a reversible 26S proteasome inhibitor used in the treatment of multiple myeloma, have been reported [48, 49]. These studies rather relate to the treatment of AMR in kidney transplantation. Woodle et al. reported promising results in this regard [49, 50]. This molecule has been used as a rescue therapy in combination with other immunotherapies for refractory AMR. Everly et al. treated refractory mixed AMR and ACR with kidney transplant recipients. They used a single cycle of bortezomib: 1.3–1.5 mg/m^2 × 4 doses over 11 days (days 1, 4, 8, and 11) [51, 52]. Alemtuzumab is a monoclonal antibody that binds to CD52 on the surface of B and T lymphocytes. It depletes mature lymphocytes without myeloablation [53]. Woodside et al. reported reversal of recurrent severe cardiac rejection [54].

A humanized monoclonal antibody against the IL-6R (tocilizumab) has been used in phase I/phase II studies for the treatment of chronic active AMR unresponsive with high-dose IVIg for patients who are difficult to desensitize. Choi et al. reported that AMR patients who had failed high-dose IVIg, rituximab, and plasmapheresis received monthly doses of tocilizumab for 6 to 18 months and they found to have good outcomes [55, 56].

Antithymocyte globulins (ATG) are antibodies directed at T-cell lymphocyte. This class of drugs is used for active treatment of ACR; thus, they are adapted for AMR treatment, but there are few data on their effect. Although there have been patients with AMR treated successfully with ATG in combination with other drugs, ATG requires more analysis as part of a randomized trial [14, 57]. Furthermore, total lymphocyte radiation is used to treat acute rejection but is risky due to its reported effects increasing hematologic malignancies [58].

Our opinion is that pAMR should be considered important due to the long-term survival of patients. If patient has pAMR, we perform plasmapheresis every other day for three sessions.

There are limited studies about treatment of subclinical AMR. Patients with subclinical AMR are not generally treated, because more data regarding the significance of a positive biopsy in the absence of symptoms are needed. Wu et al. reported that 5-year actuarial survival rates for the subclinical AMR (86%), treated AMR (68%), and control groups (79%) were not significantly different; however, patients with subclinical AMR were more likely to develop cardiac allograft vasculopathy than the control group and even tended to do worse than patients with treated symptomatic AMR [59]. The incidence of CAV or death in the patients with AMR was twice that of the control subjects [13].

Acknowledgements

The authors declare no conflicts of interest and no financial support for the research and/or authorship of this article.

Author details

Umit Kervan[1*], Dogan Emre Sert[1] and Nesrin Turan[2]

*Address all correspondence to: drukervan@yahoo.com

1 Department of Cardiovascular Surgery, Turkey Yuksek Ihtisas Hospital, Ankara, Turkey

2 Department of Pathology, Turkey Yuksek Ihtisas Hospital, Ankara, Turkey

References

[1] Stehlik J, Edwards LB, Kucheryavaya AY, et al. The registry of the International Society for Heart and Lung Transplantation: Twenty-Seventh Official Adult Heart Transplant Report-2010. The Journal of Heart and Lung Transplantation. 2010;**29**:1089-1103

[2] Boucek MM, Novick RJ, Bennett LE, Fiol B, Keck BM, Hosenpud JD. The registry of the International Society of Heart and Lung Transplantation: First Official Pediatric Report-1997. The Journal of Heart and Lung Transplantation. 1997;**16**:1189-1206

[3] Chou HW, Chi NH, Lin MH, et al. Steroid pulse therapy combined with plasmapheresis for clinically compromised patients after heart transplantation. Transplantation Proceedings. 2012;**44**(4):900-902

[4] Chaplin DD. Overview of the immune response. The Journal of Allergy and Clinical Immunology. 2010;**125**(2 Suppl. 2):S3-S23

[5] Wilson IA, Cresswell P, Davis MM, Allen PM, Trowsdale J. The humoral immune response. In: Janeway AC, Travers P, Walport M, Shlomchik, editors. Immunobiology: The Immune System in Health and Disease. 5th ed. New York: Garland Publishing; 2001. pp. 401-454

[6] Abbas AK, Lichtman AH, Pillai S. Effector mechanisms of humoral immunity. In: Cellular and Molecular Immunology. 9th ed. Philadelphia, PA: Elsevier; 2018. pp. 275-298

[7] Aranda JM Jr, Scornik JC, Normann SJ, et al. Anti-CD20 monoclonal antibody (rituximab) therapy for acute cardiac humoral rejection: A case report. Transplantation. 2002;73(6): 907-910

[8] Herskowitz A, Soule LM, Ueda K, et al. Arteriolar vasculitis on endomyocardial biopsy: A histologic predictor of poor outcome in cyclosporine-treated heart transplant recipients. The Journal of Heart Transplantation. 1987;6(3):127-136

[9] Hammond EH, Yowell RL, Nunoda S, et al. Vascular (humoral) rejection in heart transplantation: Pathologic observations and clinical implications. The Journal of Heart Transplantation. 1989;8(6):430-443

[10] Uber WE, Self SE, Van Bakel AB, Pereira NL. Acute antibody-mediated rejection following heart transplantation. American Journal of Transplantation. 2007;7(9):2064-2074

[11] McNamara D, Di Salvo T, Mathier M, et al. Left ventricular dysfunction after heart transplantation: Incidence and role of enhanced immunosuppression. The Journal of Heart and Lung Transplantation. 1996;15:506-515

[12] Loupy A, Cazes A, Guillemain R, et al. Very late heart transplant rejection is associated with microvascular injury, complement deposition and progression to cardiac allograft vasculopathy. American Journal of Transplantation. 2011;11:1478-1487

[13] Michaels PJ, Espejo ML, Kobashigawa J, et al. Humoral rejection in cardiac transplantation: Risk factors, hemodynamic consequences and relationship to transplant coronary artery disease. The Journal of Heart and Lung Transplantation. 2003;22:58-69

[14] Colvin MM, Cook JL, Chang P, et al. Antibody-mediated rejection in cardiac transplantation: Emerging knowledge in diagnosis and management: A scientific statement from the American Heart Association. Circulation. 2015;131(18):1608-1639

[15] Garces JC, Giusti S, Staffeld-Coit C, Bohorquez H, Cohen AJ, Loss GE. Antibody-mediated rejection: A review. The Ochsner Journal. 2017;17(1):46-55

[16] Olsen SL, Wagoner LE, Hammond EH, et al. Vascular rejection in heart transplantation: Clinical correlation, treatment options, and future considerations. The Journal of Heart and Lung Transplantation. 1993;12:135-142

[17] Billingham ME, Cary NR, Hammond ME, et al. A working formulation for the standardization of nomenclature in the diagnosis of heart and lung rejection: Heart Rejection Study Group: The International Society for Heart Transplantation. The Journal of Heart Transplantation. 1990;9:587-593

[18] Reed EF, Demetris AJ, Hammond E, Itescu S, Kobashigawa JA, Reinsmoen NL, Rodriguez ER, Rose M, Stewart S, Suciu-Foca N, Zeevi A, Fishbein MC, International Society for Heart and Lung Transplantation. Acute anti- body-mediated rejection of cardiac transplants. The Journal of Heart and Lung Transplantation. 2006;**25**:153-159

[19] Haas M, Sis B, Racusen LC, et al. Banff 2013 meeting report: Inclusion of c4d-negative antibody-mediated rejection and antibody-associated arterial lesions. American Journal of Transplantation. 2014;**14**(2):272-283

[20] Mayadas TN, Tsokos GC, Tsuboi N. Mechanisms of immune complex-mediated neutrophil recruitment and tissue injury. Circulation. 2009;**120**(20):2012-2024

[21] Bruckheimer EM, Fazenbaker CA, Gallagher S, et al. Antibody-dependent cell-mediated cytotoxicity effector-enhanced EphA2 agonist monoclonal antibody demonstrates potent activity against human tumors. Neoplasia. 2009;**11**(6):509-517

[22] Brasile L, Zerbe T, Rabin B, Clarke J, Abrams A, Cerilli J. Identification of the antibody to vascular endothelial cells in patients undergoing cardiac transplantation. Transplantation. 1985;**40**:672-675

[23] Mauiyyedi S, Pelle PD, Saidman S, et al. Chronic humoral rejection: Identification of antibody-mediated chronic renal allograft rejection by C4d deposits in peritubular capillaries. Journal of the American Society of Nephrology. 2001;**12**:574-582

[24] Brandle D, Joergensen J, Zenke G, Burki K, Hof RP. Contribution of donor-specific antibodies to acute allograft rejection: Evidence from B cell-deficient mice. Transplantation. 1998;**65**(11):1489-1493

[25] Baldwin WM 3rd, Samaniego-Picota M, Kasper EK, et al. Complement deposi- tion in early cardiac transplant biopsies is associated with ischemic injury and subsequent rejection episodes. Transplantation. 1999;**68**:894-900

[26] Tan CD, Sokos GG, Pidwell DJ, et al. Correlation of donor-specific antibodies, complement and its regulators with graft dysfunction in cardiac antibody-mediated rejection. American Journal of Transplantation. 2009;**9**:2075-2084

[27] Berry GJ, Angelini A, Burke MM, et al. The ISHLT working formulation for pathologic diagnosis of antibody-mediated rejection in heart transplantation: Evolution and current status (2005-2011). The Journal of Heart and Lung Transplantation. 2011;**30**:601-611

[28] Berry GJ, Burke MM, Andersen C, et al. The 2013 International Society for Heart and Lung Transplantation working formulation for the standardization of nomenclature in the pathologic diagnosis of antibody-mediated rejection in heart transplantation. The Journal of Heart and Lung Transplantation. 2013;**32**:1147-1162

[29] Ratliff NB, McMahon JT. Activation of intravascular macrophages within myocardial small vessels is a feature of acute vascular rejection in human heart transplants. The Journal of Heart and Lung Transplantation. 1995;**14**:338-345

[30] Fishbein MC, Kobashigawa J. Biopsy-negative cardiac transplant rejection: Etiology, diagnosis, and therapy. Current Opinion in Cardiology. 2004;**19**:166-169

[31] Takemoto SK, Zeevi A, Feng S. National conference to assess antibody-mediated rejection in solid organ transplantation. American Journal of Transplantation. 2004;**4**:1033-1041

[32] Kfoury AG, Hammond ME, Snow GL, et al. The Journal of Heart and Lung Transplantation. 2007;**26**(12):1264-1269

[33] Crespo-Leiro MG, Veiga-Barreiro A, Doménech N, et al. Humoral heart rejection (severe allograft dysfunction with no signs of cellular rejection or ischemia): Incidence, management, and the value of C4d for diagnosis. American Journal of Transplantation. 2005;**5**: 2560-2564

[34] Almuti K, Haythe J, Dwyer E, et al. The changing pattern of humoral rejection in cardiac transplant recipients. Transplantation. 2007;**84**(4):498-503

[35] Pajaro OE, Jaroszewski DE, Scott RL, Kalya AV, Tazelaar HD, Arabia FA. Antibody-mediated rejection in heart transplantation: Case presentation with a review of current international guidelines. Journal of Transplantation. 2011;**2011**:1-7

[36] Kobashigawa J, Crespo-Leiro MG, Ensminger SM, et al. Report from a consensus conference on antibody-mediated rejection in heart transplantation. The Journal of Heart and Lung Transplantation. 2011;**30**(3):252-269

[37] Bonnefoy-Berard N, Jean-Pierre R. Mechanisms of immunosuppression induced by antithymocyte globulins and OKT3. The Journal of Heart and Lung Transplantation. 1996; **15**:435-442

[38] Zand MS. B-cell activity of polyclonal antithymocyte globulins. Transplantation. 2006;**82**: 1387-1395

[39] Garrett HE Jr, Duvall-Seaman D, Helsley B, Groshart K. Treatment of vascular rejection with rituximab in cardiac transplantation. Journal of Heart and Lung Transplantation. 2005;**24**(9):1337-1342

[40] Kaczmarek I, Deutsch MA, Sadoni S, et al. Successful management of antibody-mediated cardiac allograft rejection with combined immunoadsorption and anti-CD20 monoclonal antibody treatment: Case report and literature review. Journal of Heart and Lung Transplantation. 2007;**26**(5):511-515

[41] Parker CJ, Kar S, Kirkpatrick P. Eculizumab. Nature Reviews Drug Discovery. 2007;**6**(7): 515-516

[42] Parker C. Eculizumab for paroxysmal nocturnal haemoglobinuria. Lancet. 2009;**373** (9665):759-767

[43] Berger M, Baldwin WM, Jordan SC. Potential roles for C1 inhibitor in transplantation. Transplantation. 2016;**100**(7):1415-1424

[44] Muller YD, Ghaleb N, Rotman S, et al. Rituximab as monotherapy for the treatment of chronic active antibody-mediated rejection after kidney transplantation. Transplant International. 2018;**31**(4):451-455

[45] Berinert [Package Insert]. Kankakee, IL: CSL Behring LLC; 2015

[46] Cinryze [Package Insert]. Lexington, MA: Shire ViroPharma, Inc.; 2014

[47] Vo AA, Zeevi A, Choi J, et al. A phase I/II placebo-controlled trial of C1-inhibitor for prevention of antibody-mediated rejection in HLA sensitized patients. Transplantation. 2015;**99**:299-308

[48] Chih S, Chruscinski A, Ross HJ, Tinckam K, Butany J, Rao V. Antibody-mediated rejection: An evolving entity in heart transplantation. Journal of Transplantation. 2012;**2012**:1-10. DOI: 10.1155/2012/210210

[49] Woodle ES, Light J, Franklin W. A multicenter prospective, collaborative evaluation of proteasome inhibition for the treatment of antibody-mediated rejection in solid organ transplantation. American Journal of Transplantation. 2011;**10**(4):159-164

[50] Walsh RC, Alloway RR, Woodle ES. Proteasome inhibition for antibody-mediated rejection. Current Opinion in Organ Transplantation. 2009;**14**(6):662-666

[51] Everly JJ, Walsh RC, Alloway RR, et al. Proteasome inhibition for antibody-mediated rejection. Curr Opin Organ Transplant 2009;**14**:662-666

[52] Everly MJ, Everly JJ, Susskind B, et al. Bortezomib provides effective therapy for antibody- and cell-mediated acute rejection. Transplantation. 2008;**86**:1754-1761

[53] Frampton JE, Wagstaff AJ. Alemtuzumab. Drugs. 2003;**63**:1229-1243

[54] Woodside KJ, Lick SD. Alemtuzumab(Campath 1H) as successful salvage therapy for recurrent steroid-resistant heart transplant rejection. The Journal of Heart and Lung Transplantation. 2007;**26**:750-752

[55] Choi J, Aubert O, Vo A, et al. Assessment of tocilizumab (anti-IL-6 receptor monoclonal) as a potential treatment for chronic antibody mediated rejection and transplant glomerulopathy in HLA sensitized renal allograft recipients. American Journal of Transplantation. 2017;**17**:2381-2389

[56] Montgomery RA, Loupy A, Dl S. Antibody-mediated rejection: New approaches in prevention and management. American Journal of Transplantation. 2018;**18**(Suppl. 3):3-17. DOI: 10.1111/ajt.14584

[57] Hammond EA, Yowell RL, Greenwood J, et al. Prevention of adverse clinical outcome after cardiac transplant patients for murine monoclonal CD3 antibody (OKT3) sensitization. Transplantation. 1993;**55**:1061-1063

[58] Salter SP, Salter MM, Kirklin JK, Bourge RC, Naftel DC. Total lymphoid irradiation in the treatment of early or recurrent heart transplant rejection. International Journal of Radiation Oncology Biology Physics. 1995;**33**(1):83-88

[59] Wu G, Kobashigawa J, Fishbein M, et al. Asymptomatic antibody-mediated rejection after heart transplantation predicts poor outcomes. The Journal of Heart and Lung Transplantation. 2009;**28**:417-422

7

Role of Short-Term Percutaneous Mechanical Circulatory Support Devices as Bridge-to-Heart Transplantation

Ahmet Dolapoglu, Eyup Avci and Ahmet Celik

Abstract

Cardiogenic shock is a life-threatening condition and mortality remains high if there is no response with medical therapy. Recently, short-term percutaneous mechanical circulatory support (pMCS) devices have increased in use for refractory cardiogenic shock. These devices can provide full treatment or bridging to long-term MCS devices if patients need long-term support. There are four types of well-known MCS devices including Impella (Abiomed, Danvers, MA), TandemHeart (CardiacAssist, Pittsburgh, PA), and extracorporeal membrane oxygenation (ECMO) and intra-aortic balloon pump for short-term and percutaneous application. In this chapter, we aim to discuss the physiologic concept, clinical evidences and applications, indications-contraindications, complications, and comparison of these most commonly used short-term pMCS devices for advanced heart failure.

Keywords: cardiogenic shock, mechanical circulatory support, intra-aortic balloon pump

1. Introduction

Orthotopic heart transplantation (OHT) still continues to be the gold standard treatment for advanced heart failure refractory in medical therapy [1]. However, limitations of organ donation cause rapid technological growth in the field of mechanical circulatory support. For patients who cannot have a heart transplant, another option may be a ventricular assist device (VAD). A ventricular assist device is a mechanical device implanted into the chest that helps in pumping blood from the ventricles to the body.

	IABP	Impella	TandemHeart	ECMO
Insertion time	6–22 min	11–41 min	15–45 min	15–60 min
Flow	None	2.5–5.0 L/min	4.5 L/min	5.0 L/min
MAP increase	Minimal	20–30 mmHg	36 mmHg	
PCWP reduction		−7 mmHg	−14 mmHg	
Duration of support	6 h to several weeks	6 h to several days	6 h to several days	6 h to several days
Leg ischemia	0.9%	3.9%	3.4–33%	18.8%
Bleeding	0.8%	13%	Up to 59.8%	18%

MAP: mean arterial pressure, PCWP: pulmonary capillary wedge pressure.

Table 1. The types and the characteristics of the pMCS devices.

VADs are commonly used as a temporary treatment for people waiting for a heart transplant. These devices are increasingly being used as a long-term treatment for people who have heart failure but are not eligible for a heart transplant.

The bridge-to-transplant strategy integrating with a long-term continuous-flow VAD has played a major role in providing circulatory support during the waiting period prior to transplantation.

Short-term mechanical circulatory support devices (MCS) provide good hemodynamic support for patients with cardiogenic shock and these devices are increasingly used as a bridge-to-decision in patients with refractory cardiogenic shock [2]. Short-term mechanical circulatory support devices acutely improve hemodynamic conditions.

When cardiogenic shock is refractory to medical therapy, percutaneous mechanical circulatory support (MCS) should be considered. Subsequently, these patients might be bridged to durable MCS either as a bridge-to-candidacy/transplantation or as a destination therapy.

There are three types (**Table 1**) of well-known MCS devices including Impella (Abiomed, Danvers, MA), TandemHeart (CardiacAssist, Pittsburgh, PA), and extracorporeal membrane oxygenation (ECMO), for short-term and percutaneous application. Intra-aortic balloon pump is also uses for short-term support in cardiogenic shock with percutaneous way. These various devices can aid, restore, or maintain appropriate tissue perfusion before the development of irreversible end-organ damage.

Here, we discuss the patient selection, current state, ongoing advances, and implantation techniques of these percutaneous MCS.

2. İABP

IABPs are the most widely used MCS devices since its introduction in the 1960s. The IABP is a balloon catheter, which is generally inserted into the aorta through the femoral artery (**Figure 1**). At the beginning of diastole, the balloon inflates and the device increases the coronary perfusion.

By systole, the balloon deflates and left ventricular after-load reduces and increases the cardiac output. So the pump decreases the left ventricular stroke work, myocardial oxygen requirements, and increased cardiac output. In this manner, the balloon supports the heart indirectly. Since it is easy to insert, IABP is the most widely used form of mechanical circulatory support.

The indications for IABP usage are failure to wean from cardiopulmonary bypass, cardiogenic shock, heart failure, and acute heart attack. Although IABP is mainly used for surgical patients, the pump can be used during high-risk interventional cardiology procedures.

During acute-decompensated heart failure, IABP may help in supporting a patient who is awaiting a heart transplant in initial period, but if the patients need longer time, another p-MCS device can be replaced or long-term LVAD implantation may be required because of its limited length of use.

Before 2012, the American and European guidelines supported that implantation of IABP in cardiogenic shock recommended as a class I; but, in the IABP-SHOCK II trial study, IABP was not found to be associated with reduction in 30-day mortality in cardiogenic shock [3]. American guidelines have downgraded the recommendation for usage of the IABP from Class I to IIa, and European guidelines to Class III. Both American and European guidelines endorse the usage of other mechanical-assist devices that provide more hemodynamic support.

Absolute contraindications for IABP use are aortic insufficiency, aortic dissection-aneurysm, sepsis, and severe coagulopathy. Atherosclerosis and arterial tortuosity and left ventricular outflow tract obstruction are relative contraindications for IABP placement.

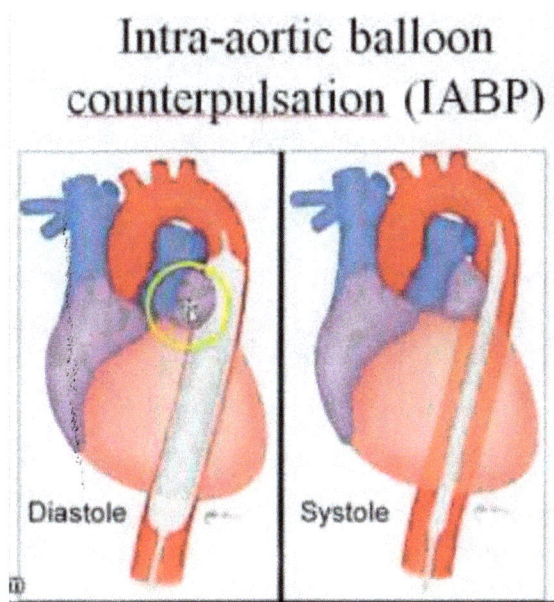

Figure 1. İABP.

3. Impella

Impella is a pump which pulls blood from the left ventricle and expels into the ascending aorta (**Figure 2**). The system has a continuous-flow microaxial pump located at the distal end of the catheter. The device can be inserted via a standard catheterization procedure through the femoral artery. It is inserted into the left ventricle via a femoral cut down or through the axillary artery, and goes through the ascending aorta, across the valve and into the left ventricle. This pump can produce a flow from 2.5 to 5.0 L/min. The principal feature mechanism of the device is to reduce the ventricular work, and to provide the circulatory support necessary to allow heart recovery.

Unlike the IABP, the Impella device uses continuous axial flow and consequently does not require pressure timing or electrocardiographic timing, allowing for stable output despite arrhythmias.

The device is mainly used during high-risk percutaneous coronary interventions (PCI) and in cardiogenic shock that is resistant to medical management. The device can also be used to hemodynamic support for the patient with severe left-ventricular dysfunction undergoing catheter ablation of hemodynamic condition [4].

In the setting of CS, two small trials have been performed with the Impella 2.5 pMCS, both using IABP therapy as the control therapy. The ISAR-SHOCK (efficacy study of LV assist device to treat patients with cardiogenic shock) trial randomized 26 patients between IABP and the Impella 2.5 in the setting of CS complicating AMI. The primary endpoint was the

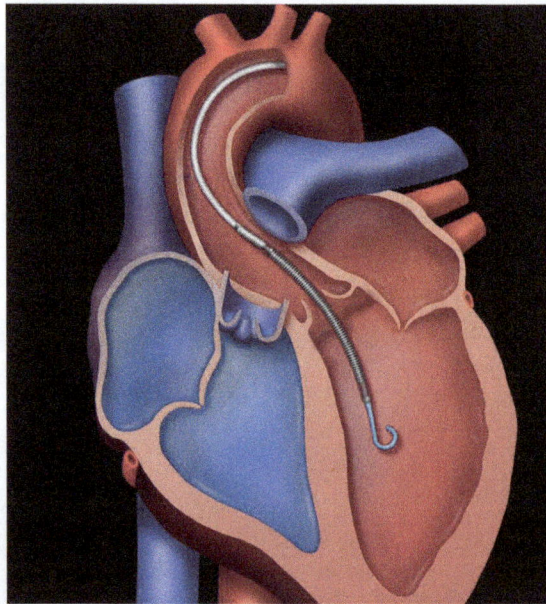

Figure 2. İmpella.

difference in cardiac index after 30 min of support, and the trial showed a higher cardiac index in patients treated with Impella than with IABP. The overall mortality was 46% in both groups [5]. The IMPRESS in STEMI trial randomized between the IABP and Impella 2.5 in patients with cardiogenic pre-shock. This study was powered for a difference in left ventricular function. However, this trial was stopped prematurely due to a lack of enrollment after 21 patients had been enrolled [6].

The Impella pump can also be used for ventricular support in patients who develop heart failure after heart surgery. The device can provide immediate support and restore the hemodynamic stability for a period of up to 7 days, and this may allow time for creating a definitive treatment strategy [7]. Hence, patients who are waiting for a donor can be supported as a bridge-to-heart transplant with Impella device.

The Impella RP is a type of Impella pump designed for the treatment of right ventricular failure that can be inserted through the femoral vein. The prospective RECOVER RIGHT study showed that the safe, easily deployed, and reliable pump resulted in good hemodynamic benefit in patients with life-threatening right heart failure [8].

The Impella pump is not appropriate in patients with mural thrombus in the left ventricle, a mechanical aortic valve, severe aortic valve stenosis or insufficiency, severe peripheral arterial disease, significant right heart failure, combined cardiorespiratory failure, and atrial or ventricular sepal defect (including post-infarct VSD).

4. TandemHeart

The TandemHeart is a continuous-flow centrifugal-assist device placed percutaneous way. Cannulas are inserted through the femoral vein and advanced across the intra-atrial septum into the left atrium (**Figure 3**). The pump withdraws oxygenated blood from the left atrium and returns to the femoral artery via arterial cannulas. The pump is capable of delivering blood flow up to 5.0 L/min.

The TandemHeart is creating a left atrial-to-femoral artery bypass that provides hemodynamic support during mainly high-risk coronary interventions and cardiogenic shock after cardiac surgery.

Among all other available percutaneous circulatory support options, only TandemHeart provides a steady supply of oxygenated blood to the body, while decompressing the left ventricle to reduce the work of the heart.

The device provides active hemodynamic support in patients who have little residual ventricular function and also can remain implanted for up to 3 weeks. For these reasons, if patients in advanced heart failure is too sick for immediate LVAD placement or transplantation, the TandemHeart may serve as a bridge-to-recovery, LVAD placement (as a bridge-to-bridge), or even transplantation.

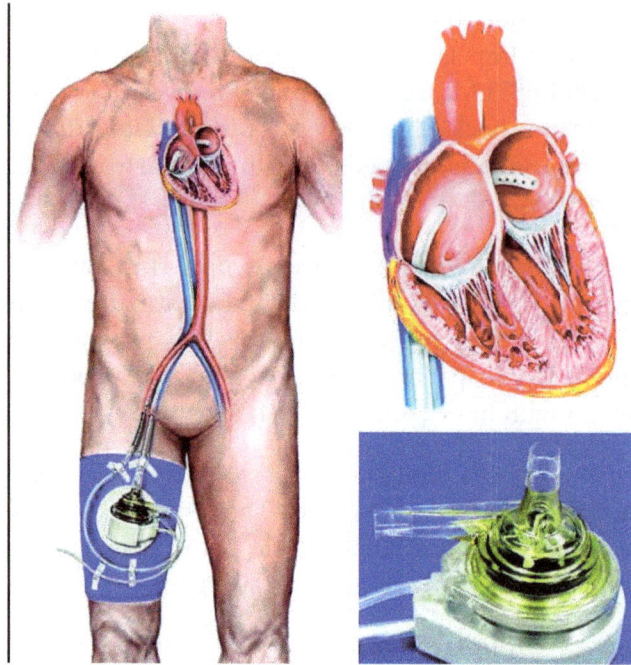

Figure 3. TandemHeart.

5. ECMO (extra corporeal membrane oxygenation)

ECMO provides a temporary support for heart and lungs. ECMO maintains gas exchange as well as cardiac support, and is used in patients suffering from respiratory failure, cardiac failure, or both. It is used for patients who have reversible cardiopulmonary failure such as advanced heart failure, acute respiratory distress syndrome (ARDS), pulmonary embolism, septic shock syndrome, and multiple organ system failure.

Blood is drained from the body with an external pump; then blood goes through a membrane gas exchanger for oxygenation and returns to the patient's circulation (**Figure 4**).

ECMO can be applied with three different ways such as veno-arterial, veno-venous, and central way. Veno-arterial (VA) ECMO drains blood from right atrium via a femoral venous or a right internal jugular venous catheter and blood returns to the aorta via femoral arterial catheter. VA-ECMO provides cardiac as well as pulmonary support. Veno-arterial ECMO (VA-ECMO) is considered in patients with cardiopulmonary collapse and is used to support patients in cardiogenic shock [9]. In non-post-cardiotomy failure patients requiring urgent cardiac support, peripheral VA-ECMO through the femoral artery and vein is the most common approach. Peripheral VA-ECMO has limitations, including retrograde blood flow leading to inadequate LV decompression. To solve this problem, some centers utilize concurrent IABP [10] or Impella [11] support to reduce the LV after-load, and hence pulmonary edema. Veno-venous (VV) ECMO drains blood from the right atrium and blood returns to the right atrium through the femoral or jugular venous catheter. VV-ECMO requires good cardiac function and mainly uses in isolated severe respiratory failure. Veno-venous ECMO is reserved for patients in isolated respiratory failure with no significant cardiac dysfunction. Central ECMO can be applied after cardiac surgery if the heart cannot be weaned from the heart-lung machine due to post-cardiotomy syndrome. Cannulas, which are inserted for heart lung machine, can be connected to the ECMO circuit and the sternum leaves open and patient can transfer to the ICU with ECMO support for healing period.

With cardiac failure, VA-ECMO is the preferred method because it provides urgent circulatory support with oxygenation in the event of sudden heart failure, thus preventing organ damage. For this reason, it may help to support a patient who is awaiting a heart transplant.

Among other devices, one advantage of ECMO is providing hemofiltration and dialysis. The connectors have been incorporated between the oxygenator outlet and pump inlet so that a continuous renal replacement therapy (CRRT) device can be attached to the extracorporeal circuit.

In a VA-ECMO setting, when the heart has recovered, but if the lungs are still poorly functioning, the native cardiac output bounces against the pumped blood, usually in the aortic arch region. Accordingly, the coronary arteries, and to a variable degree the supra-aortic vessel as well, are provided with hypoxic blood, heart, and brain are harmed. Upper extremity cyanosis has brought up the term "Harlequin syndrome." Therapeutic options consist of a relocation of the arterial cannula in to right subclavian artery or aorta, or in converting the system into a VA-V-setting.

The healthcare team looking after patients on short-term percutaneous MCS aim to avoid any complications that may occur from being on these devices. Some of the more serious problems that may occur in these patients include: (1) bleeding especially from

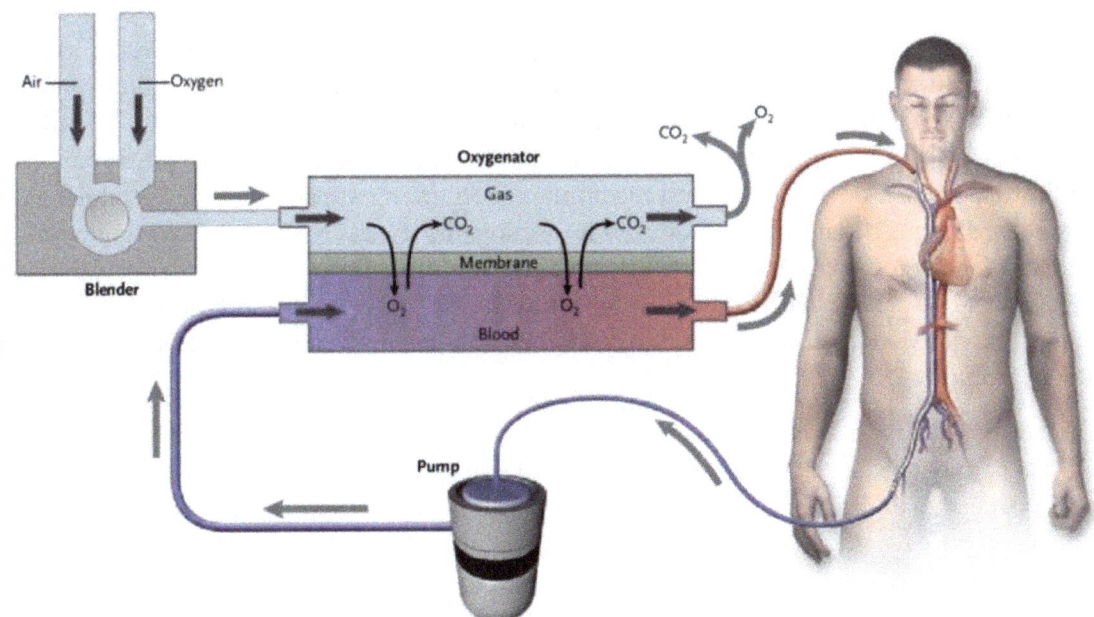

Figure 4. ECMO.

gastrointestinal system and brain. This can be a very serious problem if the bleeding happens in their brain, lungs, insertion sites of cannulae, or from gastrointestinal system. The patients should be monitored very carefully by frequent physical examinations and lab tests to make sure there is no bleeding. If there is bleeding, then medications can be given to help the blood to stop. Sometimes, surgery is needed to stop the bleeding. Blood and other blood products (such as platelets) may also need to be given if blood counts drop too low. (2) Acute renal failure may sometimes occur due to inadequate blood flow to their kidneys. With dialysis, the kidney damage may get better. However, in some cases, patients may need dialysis for the rest of their life. (3) Systemic or localized infection is another risk for these patients especiall from the insertion site. Infections in these patients can usually be treated with antibiotics. However, some infections can cause to get sick and more organ damages. (4) Leg ischemia is usually the most common problem in these patients due to insertion of the catheter or cannulas through the femoral vessels. In some cases, blood flow may be affected in lower extremity due to occlusion of the vessels and ischemia may occur. Doctors should always be aware of leg ischemia. If this happens, surgery may be needed to get blood flowing back down the leg. (5) Stroke: in patients on short-term p-MCS, stroke is another life-threating complication because of potential small blood clots. This can cause a stroke, and parts of the brain may be permanently damaged. Percutaneous MCS devices can also cause hemolysis and thrombocytopenia.

Mechanical circulatory support can prevent multi-organ failure and death in patients with advanced heart failure during waiting period. Long-term continuous-flow VAD has played a major role in providing circulatory support during the waiting period prior to transplantation, but long-term LVAD must be inserted through a thoracotomy or sternotomy, which can be hazardous and time consuming. For these reasons, patients in decompensated heart failure are best served by an initial period of stabilization with temporary devices.

Most series have combined a variety of temporary devices, but few long-term devices, and the evaluations have involved all patients with cardiogenic shock regardless of the indication for and the type of mechanical support and widely varying rates of recovery have been reported. There are four commonly used types of MCS available, which is temporary and percutaneous application. But the device choice and the implantation timing are not definitely established. Data regarding percutaneous MCS devices in cardiogenic shock are limited. A meta-analysis of three randomized trials comparing TandemHeart and Impella to IABP, TandemHeart and Impella were associated with higher cardiac index, higher mean arterial pressure, lower pulmonary capillary wedge pressure, but increased bleeding complications and no difference in 30-day mortality [12].

Another trial study showed that the Impella was not associated with decreased 30-day mortality in cardiogenic shock compared to IABP [13]. Each device should be applied according to the patient's condition and time for recovery, bridge-to-long-term devices, or bridge-to-transplantation. Another treatment strategy for percutaneous MCS is that we may consider to switch one device with other one depending on the indication. IABP can be opted for first option in patient with cardiogenic shock due to easy availability and rapid insertion. An IABP is simple and safe to insert, but provides little active hemodynamic support and depends on residual left ventricular function to be effective. If patients have worse left ventricular function, Impella, TandemHeart, or VA-ECMO can be quickly and easily inserted percutaneously and provide active hemodynamic support. During acutely depressed left-ventricular function, IABP may be the first treatment option for clinician, but if patients need more time for recovery or patients need stronger hemodynamic support IABP can switch to Impella or TandemHeart. If patients have respiratory failure along with cardiogenic shock, VA-ECMO should be opted first because it provides oxygenation and good cardiac support.

There are only limited studies available for survival of transplanted patients after percutaneous MCS. Jasseron et al. reported that transplantation was associated with a lower risk of mortality, even if the overall survival rate and 1-year post-transplant survival rate were inferior in patient on VA-ECMO and they suggested that transplantation may be considered to be an acceptable primary therapy in selected patients on VA-ECMO [14].

Percutaneous MCS can also be used for the treatment of ventricular failure in the situation of acute allograft cardiac failure or post-transplant RV failure after cardiac transplantation.

Although each percutaneous MCS device has different working mechanisms, all of them can serve as a bridge-to-bridge or bridge-to-transplant strategy. Device selection or sequential application of percutaneous MCS should be managed according to the LV function, time for recovery, and patient's conditions.

Author details

Ahmet Dolapoglu[1]*, Eyup Avci[2] and Ahmet Celik[3]

*Address all correspondence to: ahmetdolapoglu@yahoo.com

1 Balikesir Ataturk State Hospital, Cardiovascular Surgery Clinic, Balikesir, Turkey

2 Balikesir University Faculty of Medicine, Cardiology Department, Balikesir, Turkey

3 Mersin University Faculty of Medicine, Cardiology Department, Mersin, Turkey

References

[1] Jessup M, Brozena S. Heart failure. The New England Journal of Medicine. 2003;**348**: 2007-2018

[2] Lee MS, Makkar RR. Percutaneous left ventricular support devices. Cardiology Clinics. 2006;**24**:265-275. Vii

[3] Thiele H, Zeymer U, Neumann FJ, et al. Intraaortic balloon support for myocardial infarction with cardiogenic shock. The New England Journal of Medicine. 2012;**367**:1287-1296

[4] Rihal CS, Naidu SS, Givertz MM, Szeto WY, Burke JA, Kapur NK, Kern M, Garratt KN, Goldstein JA, Dimas V, Tu T. 2015 SCAI/ACC/HFSA/STS clinical expert consensus statement on the use of percutaneous mechanical circulatory support devices in cardiovascular care. Journal of the American College of Cardiology. 2015;**65**:e7-e26

[5] Seyfarth M, Sibbing D, Bauer I, et al. A randomized clinical trial to evaluate the safety and efficacy of a percutaneous left ventricular assist device versus intra-aortic balloon pumping for treatment of cardiogenic shock caused by myocardial infarction. Journal of the American College of Cardiology. 2008;**52**:1584-1588

[6] Ouweneel DM, Engstrom AE, Sjauw KD, et al. Experience from a randomized controlled trial with Impella 2.5 versus IABP in STEMI patients with cardiogenic pre-shock. Lessons learned from the IMPRESS in STEMI trial. International Journal of Cardiology. 2016;**202**:894-896

[7] Anderson MB, Goldstein J, Milano C, et al. Benefits of a novel percutaneous ventricular assist device for right heart failure: The prospective RECOVER RIGHT study of the Impella RP device. The Journal of Heart and Lung Transplantation. 2015;**34**:1549-1560

[8] Kilic A, Shukrallah BN, Whitson BA. Initiation and management of adult veno-arterial extracorporeal life support. Annals of Translational Medicine. 2017;**5**:67

[9] Garatti A, Colombo T, Russo C, et al. Left ventricular mechanical support with the Impella recover left direct microaxial blood pump: A single-center experience. Artificial Organs. 2006;**30**:523-528

[10] Bréchot N, Demondion P, Santi F, et al. Intra-aortic balloon pump protects against hydrostatic pulmonary oedema during peripheral venoarterial-extracorporeal membrane oxygenation. European Heart Journal. Acute Cardiovascular Care. Feb 2018;**7**(1):62-69. Epub 2nd Jun 2017. DOI: 10.1177/2048872617711169

[11] Koeckert MS, Jorde UP, Naka Y, et al. Impella LP 2.5 for left ventricular unloading during venoarterial extracorporeal membrane oxygenation support. Journal of Cardiac Surgery. 2011;**26**:666-668

[12] Cheng JM, den Uil CA, Hoeks SE, et al. Percutaneous left ventricular assist devices vs. intra-aortic balloon pump counterpulsation for treatment of cardiogenic shock: A meta-analysis of controlled trials. European Heart Journal. 2009;**30**:2102-2108

[13] Ouweneel DM, Eriksen E, Seyfarth M, et al. Percutaneous mechanical circulatory support versus intra-aortic balloon pump for treating cardiogenic shock: Meta analysis. Journal of the American College of Cardiology. 2017;**69**:358-360

[14] Jasseron C, Lebreton G, Cantrelle C, Legeai C, Leprince P, Flecher E, Sirinelli A, Bastien O, Dorent R. Impact of heart transplantation on survival in patients on venoarterial extracorporeal membrane oxygenation at listing in France. Transplantation. 2016;**100**(9):1979-1987

8

Heart Transplantation in the Era of the Left Ventricular Assist Devices

Michael Mazzei, Suresh Keshavamurthy,
Abul Kashem and Yoshiya Toyoda

Abstract

Orthotopic heart transplant is recognized as the gold standard for the treatment of end-stage heart disease. However, there is a perennial shortage of donor organs. Left ventricular assist devices (LVAD) represent a revolutionary tool for temporizing heart failure that is refractory to medical management until a suitable organ becomes available. This review highlights the LVAD as a tool for bridging to transplant. The history of the LVAD and its use in heart transplantation is described, as well as the current indications for use in the general heart transplant candidate as well as for selected subpopulations. It also highlights the major complications of LVAD use, advancements in the field, and selected current controversies related to the LVAD as bridge-to-transplant therapy.

Keywords: heart transplantation, ventricular assist devices, LVAD, mechanical circulatory support, bridge to transplant

1. Introduction

End-stage heart disease represents a worldwide epidemic, with over 6.6 million people affected in the United States alone. The prevalence of end-stage heart disease is increasing due the aging population in the US and Europe, as well as improved management and therefore increased survival of other cardiac diseases. It is estimated that upwards of 600,000 new cases diagnosed each year. Furthermore, the incidence of end-stage heart disease is estimated to increase at a rate of 25% by the year 2030 [1]. The disease is associated with significant morbidity and mortality; 50% of patients in this population will die within 4 years; in the subset of patients hospitalized with acute heart failure, 40% will be readmitted or die within 1 year. In suitable candidates, heart transplantation is the gold standard therapy for this disease, providing the best opportunity for long-term survival and improved quality of life. However, organs that are suitable for transplantation are a scarce resource. This approach is limited for many years by availability of donor hearts as only approximately 2300 orthotopic heart transplants are performed each year; the pool of patients who are candidates for heart transplantation continues to increase, with no evidence that this trend will reverse any time soon. As a result, the management of end-stage heart failure with cardiac transplantation must increasingly rely on an armamentarium of medical and mechanical tools for bridging patients to transplant.

In particular, the introduction of the left ventricular assist devices (LVAD) has become instrumental in the management of the heart failure patient who is refractory to medical therapy; in their current iteration their use has been associated with a decrease in mortality and an improvement in the quality of life among suitable patients awaiting transplantation. In this review, we will discuss a brief history of the LVAD as it relates to heart transplantation, in particular the evolution of available devices, and the current indications for use. It bears highlighting that LVAD implantation is associated with significant device-related complications and these are described in detail. Lastly, we will discuss several topics of current controversy and areas of evolution within the field of mechanical device support of the heart transplant candidate.

2. History

2.1. Early LVAD devices

A timeline of advances in LVAD technology and in heart transplantation is included in **Figure 1**. In the early 1950s, open-heart surgery was associated with high mortality as a result of the frequent complication of postcardiotomy shock, a problem for which there was little answer at the time. In order to combat this problem, cardiopulmonary bypass as a means of bridging to recovery became a major experimental target. Initial clinical use of a cardiopulmonary bypass system for temporary circulatory support may be attributed to the work of Gibbon in 1953. This work into circulatory support would pave the way for future innovation in development of intracorporeal left ventricular assist devices.

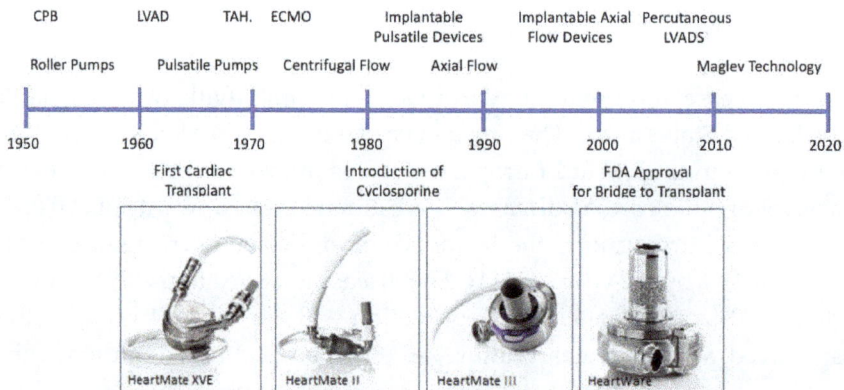

Figure 1. Timeline of advances in mechanical cardiac support and heart transplantation.

In 1964, the National Heart, Lung, and Blood Institute established the Artificial Heart Program with the express goal of developing therapies that would allow for the bridging of patients with postcardiotomy shock to recovery. Liotta and Crawford at the Texas Heart Institute are identified as performing the first LVAD implantation in 1963. The index patient was successfully weaned from the device from a cardiopulmonary standpoint; however, he ultimately succumbed to neurologic complications. Further modifications by Liotta and DeBakey led to first use of a paracorporeal LVAD for bridge to recovery after double valve replacement in a 37-year old female patient in 1966. After 10 days of support, the patient recovered and the LVAD was explanted without complication; the patient ultimately survived another 6 years prior to death due to a motor vehicle accident.

Concurrent with these initial models for mechanical circulatory support for bridge to recovery, the innovative concept of orthotopic heart transplant was also undergoing experimentation. This therapy was first demonstrated in animal models by Lower and Shumway in 1966, and subsequently the first human-to-human heart transplant performed by Barnard in 1967. With the advent of this new therapy, an alternative use for the LVAD besides bridge to recovery was identified. In 1969, Cooley implanted the first temporary total artificial heart into a patient as a bridge to cardiac donor availability for heart transplantation; his patient survived with total artificial heart support for over two and a half days prior to transplantation but died in the early postoperative period due to pneumonia. Mechanical complications associated with the total artificial heart led to a greater focus on the LVAD as preferred mechanical support after open heart surgery; in 1975 the first clinical trials of LVADs as temporary support after open-heart surgery were initiated, and in 1978, the first LVAD as bridge to transplant was used by Dr. Frazier.

Advances in technology and better understanding of cardiac flow dynamics have contributed to the evolution of the rapid VAD as a mechanical device. Early VADs made use of implanted pneumatic pump-driven volume displacement technology to drive forward flow. These first generation LVADs, mimic the function of the heart. The first generation of volume displacement pumps had multiple complex moving parts, with one-way valves and a flexible pumping chamber. Because of this, the devices were susceptible to breakdown and failure, among other complications.

The Pierce-Donachy VAD was a displacement device that was developed at Penn State University in 1970; it would serve as the prototype for Thoratec pulsatile-low VADs utilizing a pusher-plate system which could be implanted either paracorporeally (Thoratec pVAD) or intracorporeally (iVAD). This membrane-displacement technology was also used in the development of the 1978 Model 7 LVAD, later modified to the Heartmate implantable pneumatic and first used in clinical trials in 1986 [2]. A further evolution would lead to a variation known as the HeartMate VE (vented electric), and subsequently the HeartMate XVE (extended vented electric). By 1990, the FDA had given approval of LVAD as a bridge to heart transplant therapy, and a 1999 single-institution retrospective review of the use of the HeartMate XVE in bridge to transplant identified 75% of candidates as undergoing successful transplantation after a mean LVAD use of 106 days [3].

The success of LVAD as a bridge to led to clinical trials exploring the use of the LVAD as durable therapy. Perhaps the most well-known of the major clinical trial assessing the functionality of a LVADs for long-term use was the Randomized Evaluation of Mechanical Assistance for the Treatment of Congestive Heart Failure (REMATCH) trial of 2001 [4]. Here, patients with end-stage heart failure who were not candidates for heart transplantation underwent either LVAD implantation using the HeartMate VE or received maximal medical therapy; these two groups were compared for long-term complication and mortality outcomes. In this landmark study, survival among the VAD placement group was found to be 52% compared to 25% in the medical management group at 1 year, with a further 48% relative risk reduction in mortality over the 2-year study period. Additionally, the LVAD cohort was also highlighted as having improved quality of life.

However, we highlight the REMATCH study here primarily because it also identified a number of serious complications and limitations related to the use of LVAD support as durable therapy. The pulsatile flow HeartMate VE first-generation LVAD used in this study was found to have a rate of serious complications 2.35 times greater than in medical therapy group. Indeed, this group carried a relative risk of stroke 4.35 times that of the medical group. Intraperitoneal placement of the large LVAD device was associated with early satiety, and the extensive surgical dissection required for implantation was associated with a significant bleeding and infection risk. Over 21% of patients ultimately required device replacement. As a result, and primarily due to the long-term risk of infection and mechanical failure, the-year survival in the LVAD group was limited to 23% [4].

2.2. The modern era of LVAD

Continuous-flow devices making use of either an axial flow model (second-generation LVADs) or a centrifugal flow model (third-generation) were the next innovation in LVAD performance. The second generation has key mechanical advantages compared prior, including elimination of valves and chambers and the introduction of an internal rotor suspended by contact bearings. These alterations were theorized to lead to a decreased rate of complications, due in part to their fewer moving parts. However, analysis of outcomes has also shown that the direct contact between the bearings and blood in second generation LVADs serves as an area of thrombosis formation.

The second generation of LVADs were implemented into clinical practice in the late 1990's and demonstrated an acceptable safety profile for bridge to transplant when compared to existing pulsatile-flow devices despite the aforementioned higher-than-expected incidence of pump thrombosis. Approval of these later-generation LVAD's was primarily derived from three landmark clinical trials either directly comparing the pulsatile HeartMate XVE with the continuous flow HeartMate II [5], or with the use of historical controls to compare their outcomes [6, 7]. The earliest of these studies was a prospective multicenter trial of 133 patients with end-stage heart failure who underwent VAD therapy as a bridge to transplant [6]. Among these participants, a total of 100 (75%) survived to the principal aggregate outcome of either heart transplant, cardiac recovery, or survival to the end of the study; of note, of those patients on persistent mechanical support through the study, there was a 1-year survival of 67%. There was no control group in this study, but survival was compared favorably with a historical control of 53% 1-year survival among patients using the pulsatile-flow HeartMate XVE as a bridge to transplant. A follow-up study identified further improvements in survival among those using these devices, with that improvement being attributed to increased device experience [7]. Another major study evaluating the morbidity benefit of continuous over pulsatile-flow VADS identified an 1-year endpoint of stroke, reoperation, or mortality-free VAD use of 46% in the continuous flow cohort compared to 11% in the pulsatile flow cohort [5]. Further multi-center reporting of adverse events between the two groups also demonstrated a statistically significant reduction in infection, neurologic dysfunction, renal and respiratory dysfunction, and need for device replacement resulting from mechanical failure among those patients with continuous-flow LVADs.

The third generation of LVADs relies on centrifugal continuous flow. The key technological advancement in the third generation LVAD is the implementation of noncontact bearings, which utilize magnetic levitation and decrease the incidence of thrombosis due to the lack of contact. In recent years, much of the data regarding the comparative effectiveness of LVADS stems from the Interagency Registry of Mechanically Assisted Circulatory Support (INTERMACS) organization, which serves as a multi-center registry data registry. From this, we identify >20,000 patients that have been implanted with an LVAD nationwide [8]. A 2011 multicenter trial by Strueber et al. [9] identified survival rates during support in patients bridged to transplant at being 84 and 79% at 1 and 2 years post-transplant, respectively. The ADVANCE multicenter clinical trial identified greater than 86% survival at 1 year among those patients using a third generation VAD, with improved functional capacity, quality of life, and a decreased complication profile. Under a continued access protocol of the latter study, the use of third generation VADs as a bridge to transplant continues to demonstrate a high preoperative survival rate despite a low rate of transplant. Although frequent hospitalizations due to device-related issues and other complications are noted, rates of adverse event rates are similar to or improved from those observed in historical bridge-to-transplant trials, despite longer exposure times due to longer survival and lower transplant rates.

Recent advances include the approval of the HeartMate III as a bridge to transplantation. This is an intrapericardial centrifugal-flow pump making use of pump rotor that is levitated and completely suspended by magnetic forces. This is designed to minimize shear stress, stasis, and platelet activation compared to earlier LVAD models. Its unique design allows for functioning in the absence of any friction or heat generation; furthermore, it holds the capacity for device-initiated pulsatility of flow. The burgeoning evidence from clinical trials have been encouraging; results of the Conformité Européene Mark study evaluating the HeartMate IIII demonstrated a mortality rate of 18% with low rates of embolic events and no cases of pump thrombosis [10] the concurrent MOMENTUM 3 trial further supports a significantly reduced rate of bleeding or thrombotic complications among HeartMate III users, with 69% achieving complication freedom compared to 55% of HeartMate II users at 1 year [11].

3. Indications for LVAD bridge-to-transplant

3.1. Current outcomes

While left ventricular assist devices are increasingly used in the role of bridge to transplant, conflicting data exists regarding outcomes compared to the patients who proceed directly to transplant. Outcomes are improving both as a result of greater use of the continuous flow device, and as a result of more sophisticated algorithms for dealing with LVAD complications. Currently, current survival to transplant and post-transplant outcomes appear to be essentially equal between groups, especially in the absence of LVAD-related complications. Graft rejection also appears to be similar in patients who are bridged with LVADs compared to those without LVADs.

3.2. General indications

Currently, the European Society of Cardiology guidelines for treatment of end stage heart failure include the use of left ventricular assist devices as a Class IB recommendation in patient's refractory to medical therapy while waiting for a heart transplant. In addition, the American Heart Association has also issued a guidance document describing the use of mechanical circulatory support in the setting of bridge to transplant as a Class IB recommendation [12]. There is data to suggest that patients bridged to heart transplant with LVAD have higher post-transplant mortality compared to those without LVADs. However, much of this data stems from old risk calculations based on outcomes after implantation of pulsatile flow LVADs. As identified above, complication rates improved markedly as these devices have largely given way to continuous flow VADs with a more acceptable side-effect profile.

The current indications for heart transplantation include hemodynamically compromised patients with New York Heart Association class III-IV, as well as patients with stage D heart failure who are in refractory cardiogenic shock and dependent on intravenous inotropic support to maintain adequate organ perfusion. Further indications include severe angina that limits routine activity and is not amenable to revascularization, and recurrent symptomatic ventricular arrhythmias refractory to all other therapeutic modalities. Once listed, the current United Network for Organ Sharing (UNOS) organ-allocation system gives its highest transplant priority status (Status 1A) to those hospitalized patients who dependent on either inotropic medical therapy, or mechanical circulatory support such as LVAD support. UNOS designates an intermediate priority status (Status 1B) to those patients who are receiving inotropic or mechanical support at home. Patients who have infectious, bleeding, or thromboembolic complications while on VAD support may be advanced to 1A status until the time of transplantation; there is an additional discretionary option where patients with LVAD support may be advanced to Status 1A based on the decision of their transplant team and lasting for 1 month before downgrade back to 1B. Most other patients are given standard priority on the waitlist (Status 2).

In order to assist with optimal patient selection for placement of an LVAD, the INTERMACS registry has developed seven clinical profiles to identify patients. (1) Level 1 includes patients who are in critical cardiogenic shock requiring mechanical support. (2) Level 2 includes patients who are declining despite inotropic support. (3) Level 3 includes patients who are stable on inotropic support. (4) Level 4 includes patients with resting symptoms. (5) Level 5 includes patients who are intolerant to exertion. (6) Level 6 includes patients who are able to engage in limited exertion. (7) Level 7 includes patients who have advanced NYHA III heart failure. In the early years of LVAD implementation, the first two profiles (Level 1 and 2) comprised 60–80% of the LVAD candidates who were considered to be candidates for bridge to transplant. More recently, a shift has occurred in response to improved patient selection and risk stratification such that that the majority of patients implanted are now INTERMACS 3 and 4 profiles. Currently, 80% of patients who are being implanted with LVAD fall within INTERMACS Levels 2–4 [13].

A number of additional risk stratification and preoperative predictive factors have been developed to help select LVAD candidates and predict in-hospital mortality. For example, a multivariable risk score has been generated from preoperative factors of destination-therapy patients, and this highlights risk factors such as low albumin, low platelet count, abnormal liver function test or evidence of right ventricular dysfunction [14]. More recently, a risk score for LVAD patients was developed which showed that age and center experience were determinants of long-term survival [15]. While conventionally, LVAD placement is increasingly likely with increasing severity of INTERMACS profile, the ROADMAP clinical trial has shown that early implantation in lower INTERMACS profiles (4–7) outcomes are as favorable as earlier trials with improvements in quality of life [16]. Survival patterns from the UNOS database suggest that with the current LVAD technology, patients supported with LVAD support as a bridge to therapy demonstrate an improved survival while listed for heart transplantation, and the use of LVADs as a bridging strategy could potentially improve patient survival while waiting for transplantation, in turn allowing for better allocation of donor hearts [17]. Similarly, a 2016 study utilizing the United Network of Organ Sharing (UNOS) database showed those patients who underwent LVAD implantation prior to being listed for heart transplantation had improved survival compared to those who were medically managed; this survival benefit extended to those who were implanted with a LVAD while awaiting heart transplantation [18].

In general, the implementation of the VAD has led to a number of significant effects upon heart transplantation and the donor population. (1) There are now a significant number of patients with end stage heart failure who would otherwise have died while awaiting emergency transplantation, who are now surviving to have heart transplants performed under non-emergent circumstances. This has a profound effect on the pool of available donors as well as the acuity of transplant. (2) Cardiogenic shock with multi-organ dysfunction, previously an indication for emergency transplantation, is increasingly becoming a contraindication to transplantation due to the relatively poor likelihood of successful transplantation. With the option for temporization and recover without risking the high perioperative mortality and loss of scarce allografts associated with transplantation, the procedure is now being supplanted by mechanical support and then transplantation when the patients are recovered and shock is reversed. (3) The overpopulation of waitlists by patients with LVADs with acuity Status 1A who receive priority over ambulatory patients will make heart transplantation increasingly unlikely as a therapy for the treatment of ambulatory heart failure. (4) The LVAD as a bridge to transplant has allowed end stage heart failure to be treated in certain patients as an ambulatory disease in an outpatient fashion, rather than a disease requiring continued ICU management [6].

4. Selected subpopulations

In addition to the patient indications listed above, there are a number of unique subpopulations with a need for heart transplantation that would potentially benefit from LVAD as a bridging therapy. For one, mechanical circulatory support is an acceptable bridge to transplantation in pediatric patients suffering from heart failure due to structural defects. The feasibility of mechanical support as a bridge to transplantation in this subgroup has been demonstrated in single- and multi-institutional [19] case reports. For example, a small retrospective case series in 2017 of five patients who underwent VAD placement for congenital heart defects with single ventricle physiology (mean age 12), had a 60% success rate in cardiac transplantation without long-standing end organ dysfunction [20]. The factors which play into the use of mechanical support in this population are the anatomy of the initial pathology and subsequent repairs, as well as pediatric patient size, which may predispose toward the use of smaller pumps over others. This relative safety of VAD support in pediatric patients has been confirmed in retrospective review of pediatric outcomes in the United Network for Organ Sharing database [21]. In general, it is agreed that pediatric patients should be analyzed on a case-by-case basis; although the rate of postoperative complications is high, the initiation of mechanical circulatory support can allow for resolution of end-organ dysfunction and allow for aggressive pre-transplant rehabilitation.

With improved management of congenital disease, more pediatric patients are surviving into adulthood prior to transplantation; this represents a growing patient subpopulation in whom LVAD support may confer a benefit. The American Heart Association opinion paper on LVAD in adult congenital disease highlights the challenges of supporting these patients; the typical history of many prior surgical and nonsurgical interventions, as well as the complex anatomy and physiology of these patients poses a challenge in LVAD implementation. Additionally, the use of the LVAD in this population is hampered by a lack of multi-institutional data regarding selection criteria and surgical technique. It is reinforced that the ultimate goal for these patients is cardiac transplant, an intervention after which most appropriately-selected adults with congenital heart disease will have survival rivaling that of recipients [22].

One unique group that greatly benefits from LVAD placement are those individuals who do not initially meet transplant criteria. In this group, entitled, "bridge to candidacy", the LVAD may provide an opportunity to alleviate relative contraindications to transplantation, such as active smoking, poor social support, undiagnosed tumors, obesity, and advanced lung disease, whereas they would otherwise automatically exclude patients from transplantation. Several months of LVAD support can be enough time for this group to rehabilitate and become eligible for a transplant in the future. For example, one study showed the utility of LVAD implantation in patients with a body mass index (BMI) greater than 30 during the process of losing weight loss in order to become a candidate for eventual transplant [23]. Recently, laparoscopic sleeve gastrectomy has been highlighted as an option for patients who want to have cardiac transplantation after LVAD implant [24].

Additionally, patients with secondary pulmonary hypertension that is prohibitive of transplant have been shown to benefit from LVAD placement. Very high pulmonary vascular resistances fall over the course of months as the left ventricle is unloaded, allowing for future transplant candidacy.

5. Complications

5.1. Readmission

Unfortunately, although LVADs is an effective adjunct in bridging candidates to transplant, they are associated with several challenging complications. Mortality and morbidity on the heart transplant waiting list has decreased owing to the advancement of VAD technology;

candidates supported with contemporary continuous-flow LVADs have favorable waiting list outcomes. However, outcomes worsen significantly once a serious LVAD-related complication occurs. In the current era, the annual rate of readmission for LVAD patients is 65% with most occurring in the first 6 months post-implant. The causes for readmission are multifactorial, are commonly due to gastrointestinal bleeding, cardiac causes, infections, and thrombosis (**Figure 2**).

Hasin et al. reported the findings of a single-institution analysis of readmissions due to complication after the implantation of ventricular assist devices over 2 years. The major primary causes in the first 6 months were bleeding (30%, primarily gastrointestinal), cardiac (30%, with

(extrapolated from INTERMACS data)

	Pulsatile Flow		Continuous Flow, Era 1		Continuous Flow, Era 2		Ratio Pulsatile: Era 1	Ratio Pulsatile: Era 2	Ratio Era 1 : Era 2
	2006 - 2012		2008 - 2010		2011-2013				
Bleeding	630	17.28	2,643	10.57	3,867	7.79	1.63	2.22	1.36
Right heart failure	90	2.47	497	1.99	1,268	2.55	1.24	0.97	0.78
Myocardial infarction	2	0.05	21	0.08	34	0.07	0.63	0.71	1.14
Cardiac arrhythmia	254	6.96	1,355	5.41	2,056	4.14	1.29	1.68	1.31
Pericardial drainage	64	1.75	185	0.74	271	0.55	2.36	3.18	1.35
Hypertension	118	3.24	197	0.79	367	0.74	4.1	4.38	1.07
Arterial non-CNS thrombosis	14	0.38	39	0.16	93	0.19	2.38	2	0.84
Venous thrombotic event	59	1.62	191	0.76	303	0.61	2.13	2.66	1.25
Hemolysis	23	0.63	143	0.53	588	1.18	1.19	0.53	0.45
Infection	832	22.81	2,492	9.96	3,933	7.92	2.29	2.88	1.26
Neurologic dysfunction	139	3.81	469	1.88	1,086	2.19	2.03	1.74	0.86
Renal dysfunction	108	2.96	364	1.46	756	1.52	2.03	1.95	0.96
Hepatic dysfunction	48	1.32	150	0.6	324	0.65	2.2	2.03	0.92
Respiratory failure	206	5.65	689	2.75	1,338	2.69	2.05	2.1	1.02
Wound dehiscence	18	0.49	54	0.22	83	0.17	2.23	2.88	1.29
Psychiatric episode	87	2.39	297	1.19	521	1.05	2.01	2.28	1.13
Total burden	281	77.01	9,786	39.13	16,888	34.02	1.97	2.27	1.15

Figure 2. Complications rates, pulsatile versus two eras of continuous flow (extrapolated from INTERMACS Annual reports: Kirklin et. al., 2011, 2012, 2013, and 2014).

50% from heart failure and 50% from arrhythmias), infections (22%), and thrombosis (14%). During the second 6 months, readmissions decrease but after 2 years, bleeding admissions were more frequent [25]. A similar retrospective single institution review of VAD complications demonstrated that progression of the underlying cardiac disease accounted for >50% of the rehospitalizations. For LVAD factors, device infection was overwhelmingly the reason for admission (57%) [26]. As unplanned hospitalizations are common after VAD implantation, and increase as one spends more time on mechanical support, avoiding complications requires a multidisciplinary team of specialists, close postoperative follow-up, a stable home support system, and a well-educated patient population. Here we highlight a number of common complications after LVAD placement in the patient bridging to heart transplantation.

The INTERMACS annual report describes complication rates.

5.2. Gastrointestinal bleeding

One of the most common causes of admission to the hospital post-implant is gastrointestinal bleeding. In the bridge-to-transplant population, large-scale studies have estimated its overall prevalence at 22% with an event rate of 0.3 per patient-year [27]. Similar studies of complications in the bridge-to-transplant population have highlighted major bleeding episodes as occurring in 25% of the cohort, with an estimated 70% due to GI sources. Continuous flow devices have been implicated, with reduced pulsatility having been found associated with a 4-fold risk of bleeding compared to those with high pulsatility. Although the mechanisms are not fully clear, it is hypothesized that axial flow devices may predispose to increased intraluminal vessel pressure, narrowed pulse pressure, and arteriovenous dilation leading to formation of angiodysplasia. Patients on LVAD have been identified as having higher mucosal vascularity as well as abnormal vascular architecture in the intestinal submucosa. Additional risk factors of angiodysplasia formation and bleeding including older age, female sex and ischemic etiology of heart failure [27]. Lesions are primarily located in the upper GI tract, although they can be located anywhere along the length of the entire GI tract.

In this setting, initial approaches to mitigate bleeding or prevent further episodes include the reduction or discontinuation of antiplatelet agents and anticoagulants and decreases in pump speed to allow for aortic valve opening and closure. In the setting of bleeding, treatment may involve injecting or clipping of the angiodysplastic area; surgical resection of a bowel segment is reserved for emergent or refractory cases. Identifying the bleeding site may pose a challenge; in the setting of failure to reveal a bleeding source after colonoscopy and esophagogastroduodenoscopy, capsule endoscopy has been found to provide little additional diagnostic yield [28]); balloon enteroscopy appears to be more effective. Somatostatin may be an effective analogue to vasoconstrict the splanchnic bed, suppress gastric acid production and overall reduce the frequency of bleeding, and may attenuate the risk of rebleeding when administered in the outpatient setting after a bleeding event [29]. In refractory cases, heart transplantation may be the only way to restore cardiovascular physiology and ameliorate the bleeding risk.

Of note, there is a significant body of research which shows that LVAD patients develop an acquired von Willebrand factor abnormality, which results in subsequent impaired anticoagulation [30]; a recent study demonstrated a reduction in the high molecular weight multimers of the von Willebrand Factor by 30% in patients with a continuous flow LVAD [6]. In a study of patients with LVAD placement, Crow and colleagues identified that patients with bleeding had significant reductions in von Willebrand factor, ristocetin cofactor, and collagen-binding capacity compared to prior to implant, suggesting that bleeding complications after continuous flow LVAD area are function of coagulopathy on a larger scale than just von Willebrand factor consumption [31].

5.3. Stroke

While the improved flow dynamics of newer-generation LVAD technology has reduced the relative risk of stroke events associated with LVAD usage, the rate per year remains quite high. The rate varies between 4 and 10% in most studies, with some modern series highlighting an incidence to be as high as 17%. Stroke after LVAD implantation has found to be associated with a mortality that is double those of patients who stroke-free [32].

The risk of stroke remains difficult to predict in this population. A number of factors, including the type of LVAD used, differences in anticoagulation practice, and the baseline risk of the patient population appear contributory. The degree of anticoagulation necessary to prevent strokes is not fully clear. Retrospective reviews of patients on both aspirin and warfarin have not found subtherapeutic INR to be associated with a stroke, nor has reduced anti platelet been highly correlated [13]. In contrast, other studies such as the ADVANCE trial have identified non-strict adherence to anticoagulation guidelines, including INR <2 and aspirin dose of ≤81 mg, as significant risk factors. Future prospective studies will be necessary to identify the correct levels of anticoagulation and antiplatelet therapy in the LVAD patient.

The results from initial bridge-to-transplant trials identified a difference in event rates between second- and third generation VADs [34]. This is supported by more recent INTERMACS annual report notes which note that there has been a decline in the rate of thromboembolic events in recent years compared to earlier [33]. The duration of LVAD usage is correlated with increasing rate of strokes and mortality; additional contributory factors included a higher rate of stroke among patients with mean arterial pressure > 90 mmHg, a history of previous strokes, malnutrition, concomitant infection and inflammation, severity of heart failure, and prior hematological conditions [34, 35]. A recent study has identified those patients with a CHA2DS2-VASc scores greater than or equal to three at the time of implant to be associated with an 18% risk of stroke compared to 4% in the population with a score less than 3 [36]. Ultimately, although the rate rates have decreased, stroke still represents a significant cause of morbidity in the VAD patient.

Current International Society for Heart and Lung Transplant guidelines recommend evaluation of pump parameters as well as CT angiography of the head and neck for diagnosis of stroke. In the setting of hemorrhagic stroke, discontinuation or reversal of anticoagulation is advised; interventional radiology or selective thrombolytic agents may be indicated in strokes without intracranial hemorrhage [37]. In a small case series of LVAD patients with acute ischemic stroke, thrombectomy with or without thrombolytics was not associated with intracerebral hemorrhage as a complication. Therapeutic anticoagulation on an LVAD should not contraindicate thrombectomy [38].

5.4. Infection

Infection represents a major limiting factor in the LVAD patient. Post-implantation device related infection is associated with significant morbidity, raising costs and length of stay. Modern clinical trials of LVAD efficacy for bridge-to-transplant therapy reported incidence of sepsis between 20 and 44% patients-year and driveline infection of 10.7–21%, although in some cases this may be as high as 30% [39]. Recent retrospective analysis identifies a 1- and 3-year freedom from LVAD infection to be 60 and 32%, respectively. High body mass index, diabetes, malnutrition, trauma to the exit site, surgical factors, and low lymphocyte count have all been found to increase the incidence of infection. Length of implantation of the device is also implicated with longer periods of implantation being associated with increasing risk [40]. While early infection tends to present as driveline infections, late infections tend to present as bacteremia. Predictors of death in those with sepsis include presence of right ventricular failure and non-Gram-positive cocci infection. Persistent bacteremia has been found to be a predictor for further events, including strokes.

Recent retrospective analysis of the UNOS database has identified increased mortality among LVAD patients with infection. One single-institution study reported a 1-year mortality of 30% in those with driveline infections (with 50% of the patients dying from sepsis) [40]. In contrast, other small non-matched studies of the bridge-to-transplant population do not identify a statistically significant reduction in the presence of controlled infection. A retrospective analysis reported that pre-transplant driveline infections predicted post-transplant infection at former sites and led to longer length of stay without affecting survival [41]. Another retrospective analysis demonstrated that the presence of infection during the period of LVAD support did not affect post-transplant survival when compared to patients transplanted without prior use of an LVAD. We may surmise that while infection does have a negative effect on outcomes and may reduce the likelihood of transplantation, especially when refractory to treatment, it appears that selected patients with controlled LVAD infection have comparable rates of transplantation as well as early and late post-transplant survival.

Even if infection does not directly lead to morbidity at the time of transplant, there may be long-term implications; for example; the surgery may be more challenging, and there may be increased allosensitization as Class I and II panel reactive antibodies levels are higher in the device infection group. Prevention and control are therefore of paramount importance. The proper maintenance of sterility at the driveline exit site is critical; small trials have identified an absolute risk reduction of 11% after the implementation of a standardized dressing kit with silver-impregnated gauze and a standard anchoring device [42]. When infection does manifest, there is no defined treatment algorithm; treatment is often multimodal and consists of antibiotic therapy combined with local wound care, driveline replacement, and device replacement. Omentoplasty has been reported as a surgical option.

Unfortunately, conservative treatment of the infected LVAD with antibiotics therapy and local incision and drainage is not associated with clearance on infection in the majority of cases, as this approach leaves behind infected hardware; infections on prosthetic surfaces are highly resistant to antibiotic treatment due to the reduced penetration of antibiotics into biofilms. In many cases, cardiac transplantation may represent the best option for long-term survival in patients who are bridge to transplant as it represents the only procedure where all infected hardware can be removed.

5.5. Pump thrombosis

Recent INTERMACS reports and retrospective analyses note that the incidence of pump thrombosis has actually increased in the modern era, with current yearly estimates at 2.2–8.4% [43]. In 2011, there was an abrupt increase in pump thrombosis associated with the use of the HeartMate II [44]. Pump thrombosis may initially be identified by the presence of hemolysis with an increasing lactate dehydrogenase (LDH) as well as other hemolysis markers such as serum free hemoglobin and bilirubin. While the greatest risk for pump thrombosis occurs in the first 3 months after LVAD implantation, that risk continues to increase after 6 months. The risk of thrombotic device malfunction, device exchange, and mortality is greater if hemolysis occurs within 6 months post-implantation [33].

Modifiable risk factors for thrombus formation have been identified to be poor control of hypertension, suboptimal anticoagulation with a mean INR less than 2, and a lack of full-strength aspirin therapy. In modern series the pump thrombosis is associated with higher rates of tamponade, ventricular arrhythmias, hemolysis, venous thromboembolism [34], stroke, worsening renal function and poor survival. This is a lethal condition in many cases if it is not appropriately treated. Patients with pump thrombosis have a 1-year survival rate of 69% compared to 85% for patients who do not experience this complication [34]. Identification of high-risk patients remains a priority, with serial X-rays to evaluate cannula position, regular monitoring of LDH, and potentially the use of echocardiographic ramp test to detect device malfunction [45]. Additionally, pump thrombosis may be diagnosed by laboratory signs of hemolysis, evaluation of LVAD waveforms, and acoustic analysis of the pump noise.

Aggressive early intervention in patients with pump thrombosis is necessary. In a subset of patients with evidence of worsening hemolysis, heparin or bivalirudin infusion may be attempted until LDH shows a decline to normal levels and symptoms such as impaired renal function resolve. A 50–75% success rate of thrombosis resolution has been reported with this method in modern series, although bleeding events (including fatal hemorrhagic strokes) were a significant side effect [34]. A recent meta-analysis of medical management of pump thrombosis demonstrated thrombolytic therapy to be the most effective therapy at 66% salvage, but with a 20% mortality rate–albeit this was only identified when thrombolytics were used in conjunction with other anticoagulants. The use of a combination of heparin and IIB/IIIA antagonists/direct thrombin inhibitors was associated with high rates of major bleeding (35%) and intracerebral hemorrhage (18%). Death was most commonly reported after thrombolytics (20%), and the rate of intracerebral hemorrhage was 17%, but only when thrombolytics were used in combination with IIB/IIIA antagonists/direct thrombin inhibitors [46].

Often, LVAD replacement or ideally heart transplantation are appropriate management options [44]; patients that undergo pump exchange for thrombosis have a 44% mortality rate at 2 years compared to 31% after primary implant. In those with pump thrombosis who do not undergo transplantation or pump replacement, mortality may be as high as 48% [44]. A recent study found a 90-day event-free survival of 89% after device exchange compared to 60.7% after thrombolytic therapy [47].

5.6. Right heart failure

Unfortunately, the use of LVAD can be associated with concomitant worsening of right heart failure. This is defined as the need of inotropic therapy in order to support right heart function or use of right sided ventricular assist device (RVAD). Overall, right heart failure in the LVAD bridge-to-transplant population can be as high as 10–30%. This condition is associated with significant morbidity and mortality, with 71% of patients surviving to 6 months in the presence of right heart failure compared to 89% without. Furthermore, a single-institution retrospective review has identified 5-year post-transplant survival to be dramatically worse in patients who developed late right heart failure during LVAD support compared with survival in patients who do not (26% survival with right heart failure versus 87% without) Significantly worse post-transplant outcomes and increased mortality among patients with a need for both LVAD and RVAD, especially in the setting of long term outcomes, has been confirmed in large-scale retrospective database studies [48].

Identifying patients at risk for right heart failure can significantly impact candidate selection for LVAD, and has implications regarding timely and appropriate treatment, resource utilization and quality of life. Multiple pre-operative risk scores have been developed to estimate the risk of right heart failure post-implantation. Identifiers include an elevated central venous pressure/pulmonary capillary wedge pressure ratio, increased creatinine blood urea nitrogen, INR, need for and number of preoperative vasopressors, transaminitis and hyperbilirubinemia [49]. However, low sample sizes and a retrospective study design have typically limited the generalizability of these risk scores; recent validation studies of multiple right heart failure prediction models demonstrated a predictive value that was suboptimal at best [50].

5.7. Allosensitization

One issue with particular significance in the bridge-to-transplant population is that of increasing panel-reactive antibody (PRA) levels after placement of a left ventricular assist device. These devices have been shown to induce sensitization in that they are associated with the development of circulating anti-HLA antibodies with potential donor reactivity [51]. In the era of first generation LVAD support, reports indicated that these elevated levels of antibodies were linked to poorer outcomes, notably graft rejection. This association is less clear in modern studies; while some have indicated that this difference may not be significant, other studies have noted an increased level of antibody-mediated rejection in the setting of increased sensitization [52]. This remains an issue of considerable controversy.

6. Selected issues in bridge-to-transplant

6.1. Cost-effectiveness

With the changing landscape of healthcare in the United States, and a push for single-payer healthcare systems similar to that of other industrialized nations such as the United Kingdom and Canada, the clinical and cost effectiveness of bridging to transplant using LVAD bears some mention. The cost-effectiveness of LVAD support as compared to medical management with inotrope support in the bridge-to-transplant candidate has been evaluated in a number of studies.

The argument can be made against LVAD as a cost-effective treatment strategy for bridge-to-transplant. While LVAD implantation significantly increases survival compared with medical management, the survival of heart transplant candidates treated conventionally while on the waiting list has significantly improved in recent years. Therefore, the relative mortality benefit of LVAD over medical therapy has become less dramatic. Coupled with the high acquisition cost of the device, estimated in some studies to be upwards of $150,000, LVAD does not necessarily provide good value for the money spent according to established thresholds of cost-effectiveness in many single-payer systems [53].

Initial analyses based on first-generation pulsatile VADs identified LVAD support at the time as being more expensive than medical management while appearing less clinically beneficial. However, with the widespread adaptation of second and third-generation LVAD support, more recent models of cost effectiveness have identified LVAD support as delivering greater clinical benefits but at a higher cost. It remains unclear whether LVADs are clearly cost-effective from a policy standpoint, but as changes in VAD technology allow for cheaper implementation, it is hoped that cost-effectiveness benefits will become more apparent [54].

6.2. Donor allocation in the modern LVAD era

The proportion of new candidates with VADS in the heart transplant waiting list grew from 3 to 22% from 2007 to 2013 [55]. With the initiation of third-generation LVADs with continuous flow, which have fewer complications, improved durability, and smaller size, a significant improvement in survival to transplant has been realized [2]. There has been an increasing use of VADs for heart transplant over the past decade as a result of these improvements [56], and this in turn has had direct implications for the allocation of these scarce organs.

First, there is the issue of transplantation of marginal heart in the LVAD-supported candidate. The shortage of donor hearts relative to has led to the increasing use of marginal donor hearts for cardiac transplantation in an effort to increase the donor pool, as well as the increased use of left ventricular assist devices as bridge-to-transplant. Initially, propensity-matched studies of outcomes LVAD versus marginal heart transplantation have favored transplantation for better outcomes [57]. However, with the increasing validation of LVAD for extended use, the best treatment option and long-term survival outcomes remain unclear. Comparison of these populations within the UNOS database demonstrate no significant difference between waiting list survival for patients with LVAD support as a bridge-to-transplant versus survival of recipients with marginal donor hearts. Currently, this decision remains within the discretion of the transplant team and the patient, but evidence at this time suggests that there could be clinical benefits to using LVAD support in order to allow time for better allocation of optimal donor hearts as opposed to transplantation with a marginal donor heart [58].

The selectivity afforded to LVAD transplant candidates may be exposing inefficiency within the organ allocation system, which does not appear to take into account the increased survival gains made by patients bridging to transplant with LVAD. A recent study calculated a hypothetical Cardiac Allocation Score based on a number of heart failure severity stratification systems in VAD and non-VAD patients awaiting transplantation. In non-VAD patients, the majority of heart failure severity stratification scores provided accurate risk stratification; however, none of the tested scores could predict mortality among VAD-supported patients. This is in contrast to earlier evaluations that suggested that at least the INTERMACS score can provide an accurate representation of waiting list mortality in patients receiving continuous-flow LVAD support. Because the cause of death of LVAD patients is usually unrelated to heart failure; heart failure score models may either under- or overestimate the risk of mortality in these patients. This, in turn, leads to inaccurate organ allocation, and may come at the cost of detrimentally affecting the transplant chances of those patients without LVADs.

The current organ procurement protocol for patients with an LVAD is based on outcome studies performed in the era in which pulsatile flow devices were used. Based on these outcomes, patients implanted with an LVAD awaiting orthotopic heart transplant are status 1B on the waiting list, with the option of a 30-day upgrade to status 1A at the discretion of the transplant center. In addition, patients with an LVAD can be upgraded to status 1A in the event of a device complication or malfunction. However, it is not clear that patients on LVAD support necessarily merit this degree of prioritization. For example, a retrospective review of UNOS data revealed that despite being older, less favorable recipients, modern LVAD patients spend more time in Status 1A and have greater waitlist survival, which allows LVAD patients to receive preferred donor hearts and could allow for better post-transplant survival [59]. In particular, a 30-day upgrade of relatively stable LVAD patients to the highest priority level (compared with other critically ill patients at Status 1A) may allow for competition between patients with different risks of death. With this in mind, there is a concern that LVAD is perceived as a not a bridge to transplant, but a necessary gateway to transplant that is at risk of being over utilized. Furthermore, simulations have failed to demonstrate improvements in waiting list survival or post-transplant mortality with the Status 1A time allotment [60].

There is still an argument to be made, however, that the risk of VAD complications, including thrombosis, infection and sensitization that compromise post-transplant outcomes and abrogate any potential benefit that may have been realized by having the VAD; furthermore, the aforementioned allocation simulations do not demonstrate increased waiting list mortality for other candidates who did not have VADs in lieu of other mechanical support. What is perhaps the most likely reason for all of these findings is that the allocation system is already saturated with candidates at Status 1A and adding more Status 1A time for VAD patients would do little to solve the problem–instead, a more efficient method would involve risk stratification prioritization of those VAD patients at higher risk for mortality in contrast to those stable VAD patients who are at relatively lower risk.

6.3. The future of LVAD support

Studies are ongoing to develop strategies to make smaller and more durable devices, to diminish thrombosis, and to minimize surgical complication rates. A miniaturized LVAD could reduce the extent of surgical intervention, and would potentially extend the use of the LVAD for support of earlier stages of heart failure. Revolutionary future devices currently under trial will not require sternotomy or cardiopulmonary bypass; instead they will be placed through a minithoracotomy incision into a subclavicular subcutaneous pocket similar to a pacemaker. Future technology will ideally allow for completely implantable devices, as well as for devices that can provide variable flow in the LVAD, with automated modulation of flow in the setting of increased demand such as during exercise.

A return of pulsatile LVAD is also to be expected. There is recent research to suggest that pulse pressure causes vascular responses such as the endothelial production of nitric oxide and vasodilation and improved circulation in the capillary beds of end organs. Comparison of older pulsatile flow models suggest a significant hemodynamic to pulsatile flow, with increases in total cardiac output, lower pulmonary pressures, improved coronary flow, and superior left sided unloading compared to continuous flow LVADs. Based on these observations, there is now an interest in developing algorithms to generate a pulse pressure in an attempt to reduce adverse events associated with continuous flow LVADs. The HeartMate III represents an exciting disruptive technology in this regard because it holds the capacity to generate device-induced pulsatility of blood flows.

7. Conclusion

Left ventricular assist devices represent a useful adjunct in the setting of bridge to orthotopic heart transplant. There are still a number of unanswered questions regarding their efficient use; most of these questions have come about secondary to the incredible speed innovation surrounding these tools as well as their rapid and widespread adoption. There is a critical need for continued high quality studies such as large, well conducted, randomized controlled trials, particularly addressing the issues of justice in donor organ allocation, patient selection, complication avoidance, and needs of high-risk patient groups. Although this technology, and the field of heart transplantation in general, is associated with multiple remaining challenges and complications remain, it is clear that the LVAD is a powerful tool for augmenting the failing heart and stabilizing the transplant candidate while a donor organ becomes available. It represents an important facet in the holistic care of this challenging patient population.

Author details

Michael Mazzei[1], Suresh Keshavamurthy[2]*, Abul Kashem[2] and Yoshiya Toyoda[2]

*Address all correspondence to: skeshavamurthy@gmail.com

1 Department of General Surgery, Temple University Hospital, USA

2 Department of Cardiovascular Surgery, Temple University Hospital, USA

References

[1] Go AS, Mozaffarian D, Roger VL, et al. Executive summary: Heart disease and stroke statistics–2014 update: A report from the American Heart Association. Circulation. 2014;**129**: 399-410

[2] Gemmato CJ, Forrester MD, Myers TJ, Frazier OH, Cooley DA. Thirty-five years of mechanical circulatory support at the Texas Heart Institute: An updated overview. Texas Heart Institute Journal. 2005;**32**(2):168

[3] Sun BC, Catanese KA, Spanier TB, Flannery MR, Gardocki MT, Marcus LS, Levin HR, Rose EA, Oz MC. 100 long-term implantable left ventricular assist devices: The Columbia Presbyterian interim experience. The Annals of Thoracic Surgery. 1999 Aug 1; **68**(2):688-694

[4] Rose EA, Gelijns AC, Moskowitz AJ, Heitjan DF, Stevenson LW, Dembitsky W, Long JW, Ascheim DD, Tierney AR, Levitan RG, Watson JT. Long-term use of a left ventricular assist device for end-stage heart failure. New England Journal of Medicine. 2001 Nov 15;**345**(20):1435-1443

[5] Slaughter MS, Rogers JG, Milano CA, Russell SD, Conte JV, Feldman D, Sun B, Tatooles AJ, Delgado RM III, Long JW, Wozniak TC. Advanced heart failure treated with continuous-flow left ventricular assist device. New England Journal of Medicine. 2009 Dec 3;**361**(23):2241-2251

[6] Miller LW, Pagani FD, Russell SD, John R, Boyle AJ, Aaronson KD, Conte JV, Naka Y, Mancini D, Delgado RM, MacGillivray TE. Use of a continuous-flow device in patients awaiting heart transplantation. New England Journal of Medicine. 2007 Aug 30;**357**(9):885-896

[7] Pagani FD, Miller LW, Russell SD, Aaronson KD, John R, Boyle AJ, Conte JV, Bogaev RC, MacGillivray TE, Naka Y, Mancini D. Extended mechanical circulatory support with a continuous-flow rotary left ventricular assist device. Journal of the American College of Cardiology. 2009 Jul 21;**54**(4):312-321

[8] Kirklin JK, Naftel DC, Kormos RL, Stevenson LW, Pagani FD, Miller MA, Ulisney KL, Baldwin JT, Young JB. Second INTERMACS annual report: More than 1,000 primary left ventricular assist device implants. The Journal of Heart and Lung Transplantation. 2010 Jan 1;**29**(1):1-10

[9] Strueber M, O'Driscoll G, Jansz P, Khaghani A, Levy WC, Wieselthaler GM, HeartWare Investigators. Multicenter evaluation of an intrapericardial left ventricular assist system. Journal of the American College of Cardiology. 2011 Mar 22;**57**(12):1375-1382

[10] Netuka I, Sood P, Pya Y, Zimpfer D, Krabatsch T, Garbade J, Rao V, Morshuis M, Marasco S, Beyersdorf F, Damme L. Fully magnetically levitated left ventricular assist system for treating advanced HF: A multicenter study. Journal of the American College of Cardiology. 2015 Dec 15;**66**(23):2579-2589

[11] Uriel N, Colombo PC, Cleveland JC, Long JW, Salerno C, Goldstein DJ, Patel CB, Ewald GA, Tatooles AJ, Silvestry SC, John R. Hemocompatibility-related outcomes in the MOMENTUM 3 trial at 6 months: A randomized controlled study of a fully magnetically levitated pump in advanced heart failure. Circulation. 2017 May 23;**135**(21):2003-2012

[12] Peura JL, Colvin-Adams M, Francis GS, Grady KL, Hoffman TM, Jessup M, John R, Kiernan MS, Mitchell JE, O'connell JB, Pagani FD. Recommendations for the use of mechanical circulatory support: Device strategies and patient selection: A scientific statement from the American Heart Association. Circulation. 2012 Nov 27;**126**(22):2648-2667

[13] Kirklin JK, Naftel DC, Pagani FD, Kormos RL, Stevenson LW, Blume ED, Myers SL, Miller MA, Baldwin JT, Young JB. Seventh INTERMACS annual report: 15,000 patients and counting. The Journal of Heart and Lung Transplantation. 2015 Dec 1;**34**(12):1495-1504

[14] Lietz K, Long JW, Kfoury AG, Slaughter MS, Silver MA, Milano CA, Rogers JG, Naka Y, Mancini D, Miller LW. Outcomes of left ventricular assist device implantation as destination therapy in the post-REMATCH era: Implications for patient selection. Circulation. 2007 Jul 31;**116**(5):497-505

[15] Cowger J, Sundareswaran K, Rogers JG, Park SJ, Pagani FD, Bhat G, et al. Predicting sur-
      vival in patients receiving continuous flow left ventricular assist devices: The HeartMate
      II risk score. Journal of the American College of Cardiology. 2013;**61**(3):313-321

[16] Estep JD, Starling RC, Horstmanshof DA, Milano CA, Selzman CH, Shah KB, Loebe M,
      Moazami N, Long JW, Stehlik J, Kasirajan V. Risk assessment and comparative effec-
      tiveness of left ventricular assist device and medical management in ambulatory heart
      failure patients: Results from the ROADMAP study. Journal of the American College of
      Cardiology. 2015 Oct 20;**66**(16):1747-1761

[17] Trivedi JR, Cheng A, Singh R, Williams ML, Slaughter MS. Survival on the heart trans-
      plant waiting list: Impact of continuous flow left ventricular assist device as bridge to
      transplant. The Annals of Thoracic Surgery. 2014 Sep 1;**98**(3):830-834

[18] Kitada S, Schulze PC, Jin Z, Clerkin KJ, Homma S, Mancini DM. Comparison of
      early versus delayed timing of left ventricular assist device implantation as a bridge-
      to-transplantation: An analysis of the UNOS dataset. International Journal of Cardiology.
      2016 Jan 15;**203**:929-935

[19] Weinstein S, Bello R, Pizarro C, Fynn-Thompson F, Kirklin J, Guleserian K, Woods R,
      Tjossem C, Kroslowitz R, Friedmann P, Jaquiss R. The use of the Berlin Heart EXCOR
      in patients with functional single ventricle. The Journal of Thoracic and Cardiovascular
      Surgery. 2014 Feb 1;**147**(2):697-705

[20] O'Connor MJ, Rossano JW. Ventricular assist devices in children. Current Opinion in
      Cardiology. 2014 Jan 1;**29**(1):113-121

[21] Wehman B, Stafford KA, Bittle GJ, Kon ZN, Evans CF, Rajagopal K, Pietris N, Kaushal S,
      Griffith BP. Modern outcomes of mechanical circulatory support as a bridge to pediatric
      heart transplantation. The Annals of Thoracic Surgery. 2016 Jun 1;**101**(6):2321-2327

[22] Bhama JK, Shulman J, Bermudez CA, Bansal A, Ramani R, Teuteberg JJ, Shullo M,
      McNamara DM, Kormos RL, Toyoda Y. Heart transplantation for adults with congenital
      heart disease: Results in the modern era. The Journal of Heart and Lung Transplantation.
      2013 May 1;**32**(5):499-504

[23] Yanagida R, Czer LS, Mirocha J, Rafiei M, Esmailian F, Moriguchi J, Kobashigawa JA,
      Trento A. Left ventricular assist device in patients with body mass index greater than 30
      as bridge to weight loss and heart transplant candidacy. Transplantation Proceedings
      Elsevier. 2014 Dec 1;**46**(10):3575-3579

[24] Greene J, Tran T, Shope T. Sleeve gastrectomy and left ventricular assist device for heart
      transplant. JSLS: Journal of the Society of Laparoendoscopic Surgeons. 2017 Jul;**21**(3):1-6

[25] Hasin T, Marmor Y, Kremers W, Topilsky Y, Severson CJ, Schirger JA, Boilson BA,
      Clavell AL, Rodeheffer RJ, Frantz RP, Edwards BS. Readmissions after implantation of
      axial flow left ventricular assist device. Journal of the American College of Cardiology.
      2013 Jan 15;**61**(2):153-163

[26] Smedira NG, Hoercher KJ, Lima B, Mountis MM, Starling RC, Thuita L, Schmuhl DM,
      Blackstone EH. Unplanned hospital readmissions after HeartMate II implantation:
      Frequency, risk factors, and impact on resource use and survival. JACC: Heart Failure.
      2013 Feb 1;**1**(1):31-39

[27] Boyle AJ, Jorde UP, Sun B, Park SJ, Milano CA, Frazier OH, Sundareswaran KS, Farrar DJ, Russell SD, HeartMate II Clinical Investigators. Pre-operative risk factors of bleeding and stroke during left ventricular assist device support: An analysis of more than 900 HeartMate II outpatients. Journal of the American College of Cardiology. 2014 Mar 11;63(9):880-888

[28] Vaidya GN, Krease M, Dahhan A, Vijayakrishnan R, Abell T, Birks E, Abramov D. Capsule endoscopy in left ventricular assist device patients: Retrospective review of efficacy and necessity. The VAD Journal. 2017;3(1):11

[29] Shah KB, Gunda S, Emani S, Kanwar MK, Uriel N, Colombo PC, Uber PA, Sears ML, Chuang J, Farrar DJ, Brophy DF. Multicenter evaluation of octreotide as secondary prophylaxis in patients with left ventricular assist devices and gastrointestinal bleeding. Circulation: Heart Failure. 2017 Nov 1;10(11):e004500

[30] Suarez J, Patel CB, Felker GM, Becker R, Hernandez AF, Rogers JG. Mechanisms of bleeding and approach to patients with axial-flow left ventricular assist devices. Circulation: Heart Failure. 2011 Nov 1;4(6):779-784

[31] Crow S, Chen D, Milano C, Thomas W, Joyce L, Piacentino V, Sharma R, Wu J, Arepally G, Bowles D, Rogers J. Acquired von Willebrand syndrome in continuous-flow ventricular assist device recipients. The Annals of Thoracic Surgery. 2010 Oct 1;90(4):1263-1269

[32] Harvey L, Holley C, Roy SS, Eckman P, Cogswell R, Liao K, John R. Stroke after left ventricular assist device implantation: Outcomes in the continuous-flow era. The Annals of Thoracic Surgery. 2015 Aug 1;100(2):535-541

[33] Katz JN, Jensen BC, Chang PP, Myers SL, Pagani FD, Kirklin JK. A multicenter analysis of clinical hemolysis in patients supported with durable, long-term left ventricular assist device therapy. The Journal of Heart and Lung Transplantation. 2015 May 1;34(5):701-709

[34] Najjar SS, Slaughter MS, Pagani FD, Starling RC, McGee EC, Eckman P, Tatooles AJ, Moazami N, Kormos RL, Hathaway DR, Najarian KB. An analysis of pump thrombus events in patients in the HeartWare ADVANCE bridge to transplant and continued access protocol trial. The Journal of Heart and Lung Transplantation. 2014 Jan 1;33(1):23-34

[35] Kato TS, Schulze PC, Yang J, Chan E, Shahzad K, Takayama H, Uriel N, Jorde U, Farr M, Naka Y, Mancini D. Pre-operative and post-operative risk factors associated with neurologic complications in patients with advanced heart failure supported by a left ventricular assist device. The Journal of Heart and Lung Transplantation. 2012 Jan 1;31(1):1-8

[36] Koene RJ, Win S, Naksuk N, Adatya SN, Rosenbaum AN, John R, Eckman PM. HAS-BLED and CHA2DS2-VASc scores as predictors of bleeding and thrombotic risk after continuous-flow ventricular assist device implantation. Journal of Cardiac Failure. 2014 Nov 1;20(11):800-807

[37] Feldman D, Pamboukian SV, Teuteberg JJ, Birks E, Lietz K, Moore SA, Morgan JA, Arabia F, Bauman ME, Buchholz HW, Deng M. The 2013 International Society for Heart and Lung Transplantation guidelines for mechanical circulatory support: Executive summary. The Journal of Heart and Lung Transplantation. 2013 Feb 1;32(2):157-187

[38] Al-Mufti F, Bauerschmidt A, Claassen J, Meyers PM, Colombo PC, Willey JZ. Neuro-endovascular interventions for acute ischemic strokes in patients supported with left ventricular assist devices: A single-center case series and review of the literature. World Neurosurgery. 2016 Apr 1;**88**:199-204

[39] Nienaber J, Wilhelm MP, Sohail MR. Current concepts in the diagnosis and management of left ventricular assist device infections. Expert Review of Anti-infective Therapy. 2013 Feb 1;**11**(2):201-210

[40] Koval CE, Thuita L, Moazami N, Blackstone E. Evolution and impact of drive-line infection in a large cohort of continuous-flow ventricular assist device recipients. The Journal of Heart and Lung Transplantation. 2014 Nov 1;**33**(11):1164-1172

[41] Schulman AR, Martens TP, Russo MJ, Christos PJ, Gordon RJ, Lowy FD, Oz MC, Naka Y. Effect of left ventricular assist device infection on post-transplant outcomes. The Journal of Heart and Lung Transplantation. 2009 Mar 1;**28**(3):237-242

[42] Cagliostro B, Levin AP, Fried J, Stewart S, Parkis G, Mody KP, Garan AR, Topkara V, Takayama H, Naka Y, Jorde UP. Continuous-flow left ventricular assist devices and usefulness of a standardized strategy to reduce drive-line infections. The Journal of Heart and Lung Transplantation. 2016 Jan 1;**35**(1):108-114

[43] Kirklin JK, Pearce FB, Dabal RJ, Carlo WF. Mechanical circulatory support: Strategies and outcomes in pediatric congenital heart disease. Seminars in Thoracic & Cardiovascular Surgery: Pediatric Cardiac Surgery Annual Elsevier. 2014 Jan 1;**17**(1):62-68

[44] Starling RC, Moazami N, Silvestry SC, Ewald G, Rogers JG, Milano CA, Rame JE, Acker MA, Blackstone EH, Ehrlinger J, Thuita L. Unexpected abrupt increase in left ventricular assist device thrombosis. New England Journal of Medicine. 2014 Jan 2;**370**(1):33-40

[45] Fine NM, Topilsky Y, Oh JK, Hasin T, Kushwaha SS, Daly RC, Joyce LD, Stulak JM, Pereira NL, Boilson BA, Clavell AL. Role of echocardiography in patients with intravascular hemolysis due to suspected continuous-flow LVAD thrombosis. JACC: Cardiovascular Imaging. 2013 Nov 1;**6**(11):1129-1140

[46] Dang G, Epperla N, Muppidi V, Sahr N, Pan A, Simpson P, Kreuziger LB. Medical management of pump-related thrombosis in patients with continuous-flow left ventricular assist devices: A systematic review and meta-analysis. Asaio Journal. 2017 Jul 1;**63**(4):373-385

[47] Oezpeker C, Zittermann A, Ensminger S, Kizner L, Koster A, Sayin A, Schoenbrodt M, Milting H, Gummert JF, Morshuis M. Systemic thrombolysis versus device exchange for pump thrombosis management: A single-center experience. ASAIO Journal. 2016 May 1;**62**(3):246-251

[48] Taghavi S, Jayarajan SN, Komaroff E, Mangi AA. Right ventricular assist device results in worse post-transplant survival. The Journal of Heart and Lung Transplantation. 2016 Feb 1;**35**(2):236-241

[49] Kormos RL, Teuteberg JJ, Pagani FD, Russell SD, John R, Miller LW, Massey T, Milano CA, Moazami N, Sundareswaran KS, Farrar DJ. Right ventricular failure in patients with the HeartMate II continuous-flow left ventricular assist device: Incidence, risk factors,

and effect on outcomes. The Journal of Thoracic and Cardiovascular Surgery. 2010 May 1;**139**(5):1316-1324

[50] Grant AD, Smedira NG, Starling RC, Marwick TH. Independent and incremental role of quantitative right ventricular evaluation for the prediction of right ventricular failure after left ventricular assist device implantation. Journal of the American College of Cardiology. 2012 Aug 7;**60**(6):521-528

[51] Itescu S, John R. Interactions between the recipient immune system and the left ventricular assist device surface: Immunological and clinical implications. The Annals of Thoracic Surgery. 2003 Jun 1;**75**(6):S58-S65

[52] Urban M, Gazdic T, Slimackova E, Pirk J, Szarszoi O, Maly J, Netuka I. Alloimmunosensitization in left ventricular assist device recipients and impact on post transplantation outcome. ASAIO Journal. 2012 Nov 1;**58**(6):554-561

[53] Moreno SG, Novielli N, Cooper NJ. Cost-effectiveness of the implantable HeartMate II left ventricular assist device for patients awaiting heart transplantation. The Journal of Heart and Lung Transplantation. 2012 May 1;**31**(5):450-458

[54] Clarke A, Pulikottil-Jacob R, Connock M, Suri G, Kandala NB, Maheswaran H, Banner NR, Sutcliffe P. Cost-effectiveness of left ventricular assist devices (LVADs) for patients with advanced heart failure: Analysis of the British NHS bridge to transplant (BTT) program. International Journal of Cardiology. 2014 Feb 15;**171**(3):338-345

[55] Colvin-Adams M, Smith JM, Heubner BM, Skeans MA, Edwards LB, Waller CD, Callahan ER, Snyder JJ, Israni AK, Kasiske BL. OPTN/SRTR 2013 annual data report: Heart. American Journal of Transplantation. 2015 Jan 1;**15**(S2):1-28

[56] Lund LH, Edwards LB, Dipchand AI, Goldfarb S, Kucheryavaya AY, Levvey BJ, Meiser B, Rossano JW, Yusen RD, Stehlik J. The registry of the International Society for Heart and Lung Transplantation: Thirty-third adult heart transplantation report—2016; focus theme: Primary diagnostic indications for transplant. The Journal of Heart and Lung Transplantation. 2016 Oct 1;**35**(10):1158-1169

[57] Daneshmand MA, Rajagopal K, Lima B, Khorram N, Blue LJ, Lodge AJ, Hernandez AF, Rogers JG, Milano CA. Left ventricular assist device destination therapy versus extended criteria cardiac transplant. The Annals of Thoracic Surgery. 2010 Apr 1;**89**, **4**:1205-1210

[58] Schumer EM, Ising MS, Trivedi JR, Slaughter MS, Cheng A. Early outcomes with marginal donor hearts compared with left ventricular assist device support in patients with advanced heart failure. The Annals of Thoracic Surgery. 2015 Aug 1;**100**(2):522-527

[59] Taghavi S, Jayarajan SN, Komaroff E, Mangi AA. Continuous flow left ventricular assist device technology has influenced wait times and affected donor allocation in cardiac transplantation. The Journal of Thoracic and Cardiovascular Surgery. 2014 Jun 1;**147**(6):1966-1971

[60] Barr ML, Taylor DO. Changes in donor heart allocation in the United States without fundamental changes in the system: Rearranging deck chairs and elephants in the room. American Journal of Transplantation. 2015 Jan 1;**15**(1):7-9

9

Surgical Management for Advanced Heart Failure in Adults with Congenital Heart Disease

Crystal L. Valadon, Erin M. Schumer and
Mark S. Slaughter

Abstract

Adults with congenital heart disease (ACHD) have emerged as a new patient population that poses a variety of treatment and management obstacles. This chapter discusses the diagnosis of heart failure and treatment challenges faced by ACHD specifically addressing when to initiate mechanical circulatory support versus heart transplantation. It is evident that the ACHD population presents with a variety of unique challenges and considerations that still need to be explored. Addressing each of these issues will vastly change and improve how ACHD patients are approached from a treatment standpoint and ultimately provide more advantageous clinical options that can successfully handle the complexities presented by this population.

Keywords: transplant, VADs, heart failure, congenital heart disease

1. Introduction

Over the past several decades, adults with congenital heart disease (ACHD) have emerged as a new type of patient population that poses a variety of treatment and management obstacles. In North America alone, the prevalence of ACHD is estimated to be greater than 1 million patients [1]. The emergence of this group can be attributed to the clinical advancements that have been made in addressing these congenital disorders as they present during childhood and has enabled over 85% of children diagnosed with CHD to survive to adulthood [2]. As these patients progress into adulthood, they continue to experience complications and medical complexities associated with their CHD. The dominant complication that the ACHD population faces is the development of heart failure, and this is currently recognized as the leading cause of death for ACHD patients [3].

In current medical practice, the gold standard for treating end stage heart failure is heart transplantation. This however remains a treatment option that is limited by donor supply. For the past several decades, the number of heart transplants that have been performed annually in the United States is between 2000 and 2500 [4]. This supply does not meet the current demands of the growing heart failure population. As the prevalence of heart failure in the ACHD population grows, the demand for heart failure treatment will continue to increase, placing further strain on the already overburdened transplant system.

In addition to the concerns associated with donor supply, ACHD patients face further burdens when seeking heart transplantation as a treatment option due to their medical complexities that are not currently accounted for in the guidelines established by UNOS. These include younger age, anatomical complexities, and decreased likelihood of an implanted mechanical assist device in comparison to the non-ACHD candidates. This, in turn, leads to a lower urgency status, longer waitlist times, and a higher incidence of ACHD patients experiencing delisting due to clinical deterioration [5].

It is evident that further evaluation of the growing ACHD population is necessary in order to provide effective management plans for the treatment of heart failure that will account for their complex circumstances. This chapter discusses current medical management, associated treatment outcomes, and future directions in the management of ACHD patients.

2. Diagnosis

The diagnosis of heart failure in ACHD is often difficult because this population may present with atypical signs and symptoms; however, diagnosis is facilitated by regular follow-up including history and physical exam, laboratory and imaging studies, and functional testing that is part of the management of these patients. Once a hemodynamic lesion is identified on imaging, correction of the lesion is usually required. If no hemodynamic lesion is present, patients are classified into two groups based on whether or not there is impaired ventricular function. Medical management of heart failure is indicated when there is impaired ventricular function without a significant hemodynamic lesion or for patients with normal ventricular function who are clinically symptomatic with either an elevated BNP or evidence of impairment of cardiopulmonary exercise testing. Regular follow-up is indicated if BNP or exercise testing is normal or for clinically, asymptomatic patients with normal ventricular function [1].

3. Treatment

3.1. Medical management

Once heart failure is recognized, medical treatment consists of a cocktail of medications including diuretics, beta blockers, renin-angiotensin-aldosterone system blockers, mineralocorticoid receptor antagonists, digoxin, pulmonary vasodilators, calcium channel blockers, and afterload reducing agents, similar to adult-onset heart failure [1]. Treatment is tailored based on specific physiology and is outside the scope of this chapter. Other interventions include implantation of a cardioverter defibrillator [6] and cardiac resynchronization therapy [7].

3.2. Surgical management

Structural intervention is often required in patients with adult CHD and ranges from catheter based therapy to heart transplantation depending on the etiology of CHD and presentation of symptoms in adulthood. The decision to undertake surgical correction must be weighed carefully against medical management as survival decreases with an increase in the number of sternotomies [8]. Additionally, the use of blood products may cause HLA sensitization, impacting the potential for later heart transplant [9]. Cardiac surgery includes pulmonary valve/conduit replacement, closure of atrial septal defects, aortic procedures, repair/revision of tetralogy of Fallot, conversion to or revision of Fontan repair, and other valvular repair/replacements [10].

Mechanical circulatory support (MCS) assistance may be indicated for patients who develop acute heart failure resistant to maximal medical management. Extracorporeal membrane oxygenation is considered for patients who develop cardiogenic shock and often serves as a "bridge to decision" therapy in this patient population [11]. Unlike standard heart failure, ECMO is particularly useful for CHD patients who develop right ventricular failure [12]. The use of ECMO should be limited to patients who have not developed multi-organ failure as prognosis is poor in this population.

The number of chronic ventricular assist device implantations continues to increase although concentrated to relatively few centers [13]. Few patients with single ventricle morphology are implanted as most patients are classified as systemic morphological left or right ventricle [13]. Similar to ECMO therapy, long-term MCS is used as a bridge to transplant or candidacy and seldom used as destination therapy [13]. Most patients are implanted with a left VAD, but there is a higher proportion of patients compared to the acquired heart failure population who require biventricular support with either biventricular VADs or a total artificial heart [13]. Across all morphologies, axial, continuous flow pumps are more commonly used; however, there is a larger proportion of pulsatile pumps used in the ACHD population compared with those with acquired heart failure [13].

Heart transplantation is considered when estimated 1-year survival is less than 80%. The decision to list for heart transplant is complex, more so than patients with acquired heart failure, and factors influencing this decision include anatomical considerations, presence of non-heart end-stage organ failure, progressive cyanosis, degree of pulmonary hypertension, and cardiopulmonary exercise testing [14]. Patients with single ventricle morphology present particular anatomical and vascular challenges, as they often require additional surgical procedures at the time of transplant including pulmonary artery and abnormal systemic venous return reconstruction. Overall, patient selection is crucial for the success of heart transplant in adults with congenital heart disease.

4. Current outcomes for adults with congenital heart disease

4.1. Mechanical circulatory support

In the treatment of heart failure, the emergence of mechanical circulatory assist devices has become a widely accepted option for individuals who either do not meet the transplant criteria or as a bridge to transplantation. Despite their widespread use in non-ACHD patients, mechanical circulatory assist devices are not as easily applied to the ACHD population because many of these patients present with anatomical challenges such as single ventricles, vascular reconstruction of major arteries, and systemic right ventricles [2]. The complexity of anatomical variants in addition to the presence of comorbidities contributes to a higher perioperative complication rate compared with the non-ACHD population. These adverse events include higher rates of hepatic dysfunction, respiratory failure, renal dysfunction requiring dialysis, and sustained cardiac arrhythmias [13]. When compared with a matched non-ACHD cohort, Cedars et al. found that early survival in the first 5 months post-implantation was worse in the ACHD population but comparable thereafter, and functional status and quality of life parameters were similar in both groups. They attributed these findings to the operative and perioperative factors unique to the ACHD population, particularly anatomic issues and increased likelihood of having previous sternotomies. Overall, results suggest that MCS is a good option for ACHD patients with advanced heart failure despite increased peri-operative complications and mortality as a bridge to transplant and may be a viable option as destination therapy in the future. Outcomes after MCS implantation are shown in **Table 1**.

4.2. Transplantation

ACHD patients experience a variety of disadvantages when seeking transplantation as a treatment for their heart failure. Issues such as anatomical concerns and immune status can impact their ability for transplant candidacy significantly. If these factors do not influence their ability to be placed on the transplant registry, the ACHD population experiences a higher waitlist mortality than non-ACHD patients. This can be attributed to factors such as ACHD patients typically being of a younger age and less likely to utilize mechanical circulatory assist devices due to clinical barriers. As a result, they may experience longer wait list periods, a greater incidence of death while waiting for a transplant, or delisting [5].

The outcomes for ACHD patients that are successfully transplanted vary depending on short-term versus long-term comparisons and are shown in **Table 2**. Short-term outcomes for ACHD patients, similar to outcomes after MCS, are worse than when compared to non-ACHD patients: 20–30% mortality at 30 days mortality [1]. This increased mortality rate can potentially be explained by unique challenges associated with the ACHD population such as anatomical concerns and longer times of ischemia during surgery due to the need for reconstruction during the transplant [15]. One study by Paniagua Martn et al. [16] suggests that the cause for this difference can be attributed to a higher incidence of primary graft failure in ACHD patients. Despite increased peri-operative mortality, the long-term survival for ACHD patients is outstanding, with a median survival of greater than 20 years [2].

Source	Study description	Purpose	Results
VanderPluym et al. [13]	Data entered into the Interagency Registry for Mechanically Assisted Circulatory Support (INTERMACS) from June 2006 to December 2015 was utilized. The 126 ACHD patients were categorized as follows: 63 systemic morphologic left ventricle, 45 systemic morphologic right ventricle, and 17 single ventricle.	To compare mortality between ACHD and non ACHD patients after device implantation.	The survival rate was similar between ACHD and non-ACHD patients with LVAD's.
Maly et al. [17]	Five adult patients with systemic right ventricular failure after a Mustard operation were implanted with a HeartMate II VAD.	To collect data on utilizing LVAD's as bridge to transplantation devices in patients with previously palliated transposition of great arteries.	Heart failure symptoms improved in all patients; therefore, a VAD may be a suitable treatment option in bridge to transplant for patients who are severely ill.
Everitt et al. [18]	An analysis of 9722 adults, 314 of which were diagnoses with ACHD was conducted to identify key differences in listing status and outcomes.	To analyze waitlist outcomes for ACHD versus non ACHD patients in heart transplantation.	Adults with CHD were much less likely to have a VAD (5 versus 14%) and were more likely to be given a lower urgency status. These patients were also more likely to experience cardiovascular related death with waiting to undergo heart transplantation (60 versus 40%). The utilization of VAD's should be explored to determine if survival for ACHD patients can be improved.
Shah et al. [19]	A retrospective analysis of six ACHD patients who underwent VAD implantation.	To provide data for ACHD patients with VAD implantation.	Five patients survived to discharge: one patient was successfully transplanted, one patient survived 262 days; one patient received 988 days of therapy while awaiting transplantation as of December 1, 2012; and two patients who received VADs as destination therapy received 577 and 493 days and were still alive as of December 1, 2012. VAD implantation is a viable option for therapy in ACHD patients in either bridge to transplant or bridge to destination therapy.
Newcomb et al. [20]	An ACHD patient with failing Fontan circulation was implanted with an LVAD device and went on to have a successful heart transplantation 5 months later.	A case study that discusses the outcome of an LVAD implantation in an ACHD patient with a failing Fontan circulation as bridge to transplant therapy.	This case report suggests that LVAD's can become useful in patients with ACHD, particularly those with failing Fontan circulation as either bridge to transplant or bridge to destination therapy.

Source	Study description	Purpose	Results
Morris et al. [21]	A presentation of a case in which LVAD implantation was utilized as therapy option in an ACHD patient that presented with failure of the systemic ventricle.	A case study of LVAD implantation in an ACHD patient.	Utilization of the LVAD therapy significantly improved the patients cyanosis and ventricular function. This suggests that patients with ACHD could benefit from utilizing LVAD therapy.
Stewart et al. [22]	Two ACHD patients were successfully bridged to transplantation utilizing LVAD therapy. Their deterioration leading to the need for transplant can be attributed to their deteriorating right ventricular failure.	To explain the case reports of two ACHD patients who received LVAD bridge to transplant therapy.	This report suggests that LVAD therapy is a viable option for bridge to transplantation in ACHD patients that present with right ventricular failure.
Gelow et al. [23]	A retrospective study of 1250 ACHD patients reported in the UNOS database from 1985 to 2010 in which these patients were compared to non –ACHD patients in terms of VAD use at listing, listing status, status upgrades and reasons for upgrades.	To determine the relationship that exists between VAD implantation and successful transplantation in patients that are listed for heart transplant.	It was noted that the use of VAD's in ACHD patient was less at both the time of listing and transplantation. This decreased usage of VAD therapy in ACHD patients contributes to lower listing status and organ allocation.
Joyce et al. [24]	Three adult patients that had congenitally corrected transposition of the great arteries underwent LVAD implantation as a therapy option for their end stage heart failure.	A case report of three ACHD patients that underwent LVAD implantation.	LVAD implantation can be successfully completed in ACHD patients when placed under echocardiographic guidance. This offers an additional therapy option for ACHD patients.
Maxwell et al. [25]	Data collected from September 1987 to September 2012 by the Scientific Registry of Transplant Recipients was utilized to compare the following between MCS and non-MCS ACHD patient populations: procedural, outcome and survival.	To analyze the pretransplant effects of mechanical circulatory support on posttransplant outcomes in the ACHD population.	In the ACHD patient population, those with MCS are associated with higher transfusion rates and length of stay however, they do not have less favorable outcomes post-transplant when compared to non-MCS ACHD patients.

Table 1. Outcomes after mechanical circulatory support device implantation in adults with congenital heart disease.

Source	Sample/study description	Purpose	Results
Irving et al. [26]	Outcomes were reviewed from 38 cardiac transplants performed in 37 patients from 1988 to 2009 using medical records and transplant databases. 41% had univentricular and 59% had biventricular physiology.	To explore data on outcomes of cardiac transplantation in the ACHD patient group.	Operative mortality for ACHD patients following cardiac transplantation is higher than for other diagnostic groups. However, long term survival is noted to be good and comparable to non ACHD patients.

Source	Sample/study description	Purpose	Results
Patel et al. [27]	Data reported to UNOS from 1987 to 2006 was reviewed and categorized to compare adults with CHD versus other diagnoses in heart transplantations. 2% of the individuals in this study period had CHD.	To evaluate the post transplantation prognosis in adults with CHD.	The 30-day mortality rate is elevated in the ACHD population: 16 versus 6%. However, there is not a statistical significance in the 5 and 10-year survival rates for ACHD patients in comparison to non-ACHD patients.
Taylor et al. [28]	Data from heart transplantations performed from 2001 to 2003 was utilized to calculate survival rates by the Kaplan–Meier method. Adults with CHD represented 2.7% of the cohort.	To evaluate the survival outcomes for patients post heart transplantation.	Having a diagnosis of ACHD is one of the most powerful predictors of 1-year mortality. But at 10 years it is associated with a marked survival advantage conditional on a 3-year survival independent of age.
Lamour et al. [29]	The post-transplantation outcomes for 24 adults with CHD were analyzed utilizing the Kaplan–Meier statistical method to estimate survival functions for patients with CHD versus all others and patients with CHD versus matched controls.	To analyze the survival rate of adult patients with CHD post cardiac transplantation in comparison in those without CHD.	The survival rate for patients with ACHD post-transplantation was 79% at 1 year and 60% at 5 years. A difference between this population and the control populations was not present.
Davies et al. [8]	A retrospective study of patients listed for primary transplantation between 1995 and 2009 was conducted. 2.5% of these patients were adults with CHD.	To evaluate the survival of adults with CHD after listing and transplantation.	The early mortality rate (30 day) among ACHD patients was high (reoperation 18.9 versus 9.6%; nonreoperation 16.6 versus 6.3%), but at 10 years the survival rate was equivalent with non-ACHD patients (53.8 versus 53.6%)
Bhama et al. [30]	A retrospective analysis was conducted from January 2001 to February 2011. 19 patients with ACHD were compared to 428 patients with non-ACHD who underwent transplantation.	To evaluate the survival outcomes of cardiac transplantation in adults with CHD in a contemporary cohort.	There was no significant difference in survival of ACHD versus non-ACHD at 30 days (89 versus 92%), 1 year (84 versus 86%), or 5 years (70 versus 72%).
Karamlou et al. [31]	A review of heart transplantation patients from 1990 to 2008 reported to UNOS was conducted. A total of 8496 patients were evaluated, of which 575 had ACHD.	To investigate outcomes and risk factors for mortality and retransplantation for the ACHD population in comparison to the non-ACHD population.	The overall post-transplantation mortality and retransplantation rates were significantly higher for patients with ACHD mainly due to an early hazard phase.
Burchill et al. [32]	A retrospective study was conducted on patients who were identified in the registry of ISHLT between 1985 and 2010. The Kaplan–Meier method was used to conduct a survival comparison. 2.2% of patients transplanted in this cohort had a diagnosis of ACHD.	To examine survival, causes of death and predictors of early (<1 year), mid-term (1–5 years) and later (0.5 years) mortality in ACHD patients who received cardiac transplants.	Early mortality rates for the ACHD population was high in comparison to the non-ACHD transplant recipients (10 versus 4%). The long-term survival rates for ACHD patients who survived the early hazard phase was superior to the non-ACHD patients.

Source	Sample/study description	Purpose	Results
Paniagua Martin et al. [16]	Survival outcomes in a total of 3166 patients were included: 1888 IHD, 1223 IDCM, and 55 ACHD.	To analyze the survival probability between different subgroups with ACHD.	The early mortality rating associated with ACHD can primarily be attributed to the presence of primary graft failure. The frequency of primary graft failure in ACHD was 23%, versus 17% in IHD and 13% in IDCM. The following is the frequency of early mortality rates: 25% CHD, 14% IDCM, 16% IHD.
Singh et al. [33]	Adults who underwent heart transplantation in the United States between January 2007 and June 2009 were utilized to determine and validate the risk prediction model. This efficiency of this model was further assessed by evaluating the performance in patients from July 2009 to October 2010 receiving heart transplants.	To develop a risk prediction model for posttransplant in hospital mortality in heart transplant patients.	The model determined that the ACHD diagnosis is correlated with an odds ratio of 4.18 for early in hospital mortality post heart transplantation.
Karamlou et al. [34]	A comparison among in hospital deaths between ACHD patients that possessed either 1 V or 2 V anatomy was conducted retrospectively from 1993 to 2007 through data gathered in the Nationwide Inpatient Sample (NIS).	To determine if there is an associated with early death post heart transplantation in patients who possess 1 V anatomy in ACHD.	ACHD patients that possess 1 V anatomy are associated with a higher death incidence post heart transplantation. Transplantation registries should include specific ACHD diagnoses due to the evident difference in associated outcomes.

Table 2. Outcomes after heart transplantation in adults with congenital heart disease.

Regardless of this data, outcomes for patients with ACHD after transplantation vary depending on their initial diagnosis. As there are a variety of clinical manifestations of ACHD, assessing prognostic values remains challenging and therefore individuals should be evaluated thoroughly prior to transplant consideration.

5. Conclusion

Further investigation into the ACHD population is essential in order to effectively manage their unique medical concerns as this patient group continues to expand. This investigation must occur from multiple points in order to ensure the variety of distinct challenges presented by this population are adequately addressed. Specifically, there are four areas this chapter suggests future research efforts should focus on in order to provide the most advantageous information for medical management:

- The cause of increased early mortality rates in heart transplant operations for ACHD patients. After thorough review of the current literature, it is evident that ACHD patients experience higher early mortality rate post heart transplantation in comparison to non-ACHD patients. However, at this point in time little research has been focused on identifying the clinical source for this mortality contrast. It is essential that research efforts focus on seeking out the root of this disparity in order to work towards minimizing the presence of this current complex outcome. Doing so will supply the medical community with more accurate predictors of mortality when seeking heart transplantation as treatment for these patients and provide better outcomes to those who undergo this type of medical management.

- Determining the appropriate timing/type of interventions to utilize for this clinically diverse group. Due to the clinical diversity that exists within the ACHD patient populations applying standardized treatment regimens remains challenging. Case studies exploring how to effectively manage different anatomical morphologies currently exist but this aspect of research still remains relatively unexamined and information specifically regarding timing is rather limited. Increasing the knowledge in terms of how to effectively approach treatment in ACHD patients in terms of when and how to intervene will assist in decreasing the complexity of approaching a therapy regimen and provide stronger evidence to provide the best possible clinical outcomes for these patients.

- Re-evaluating how ACHD patients are listed into the transplant registries. With the current listing guidelines ACHD patients are at a significant disadvantage in terms of their likelihood of being successfully transplanted. As of now, ACHD patients are more likely to experience a lower listing status with their initial listing than non-ACHD patients. In addition, ACHD patients experience a high rate of delisting after 1 year due to a decline in their worsening condition. These patients are placed at an even further disadvantage because they may not be candidates for mechanical circulatory support due to anatomical constraints. Therefore, they are unable to utilize the placement of these devices to prolong their survival to successfully reach transplantation, or utilize the benefits of attaining a higher listing status associated with these interventional therapies. The current listing criteria for heart transplantation is a cause of serious concern when considering ethical and effective medical management for patients with ACHD. There is an urgent need for re-evaluation of these current guidelines to occur in order to take into consideration the unique medical challenges presented by this growing population that will continue to rely on heart transplantation as one of their main treatment possibilities in the future.

- Exploring the use of MCS as destination therapy in addition to bridge to transplantation. The utilization of these devices for treatment in ACHD patients has previously focused on their usage as bridge to transplant therapy. However, with the increasing demand for heart transplantation, it is imperative that other therapy options are considered for ACHD patients. More recently, the use of MCS has been considered as destination therapy for this group of patients. Current research indicates that there is potential for pursuing this line of treatment option for a variety of ACHD subgroups. Doing so would provide an effective treatment option for these patients and relieve some of the current burden on the transplant system.

It is evident that the ACHD population presents with a variety of unique challenges and considerations that still need to be explored. Addressing each of these areas mentioned above will vastly change and improve how ACHD patients are approached from a treatment stand-point and ultimately provide more advantageous clinical options that can successfully handle the complexities presented by this population.

Author details

Crystal L. Valadon, Erin M. Schumer and Mark S. Slaughter*

*Address all correspondence to: mark.slaughter@louisville.edu

Department of Cardiovascular and Thoracic Surgery, University of Louisville, Kentucky, USA

References

[1] Budts W, Roos-Hesselink J, Radle-Hurst T, et al. Treatment of heart failure in adult congenital heart disease: A position paper of the Working Group of Grown-Up Congenital Heart Disease and the Heart Failure Association of the European Society of Cardiology. European Heart Journal. 2016;**37**:1419-1427

[2] Gurvitz M, Burns KM, Brindis R, et al. Emerging research directions in adult congenital heart disease: A report from an NHLBI/ACHA Working Group. Journal of the American College of Cardiology. 2016;**67**:1956-1964

[3] Van De Bruaene A, Hickey EJ, Kovacs AH, et al. Phenotype, management and predictors of outcome in a large cohort of adult congenital heart disease patients with heart failure. International Journal of Cardiology. 2018;**252**:80-87

[4] Kilic A, Emani S, Sai-Sudhakar CB, Higgins RS, Whitson BA. Donor selection in heart transplantation. Journal of Thoracic Disease. 2014;**6**:1097-1104

[5] Matsuda H, Ichikawa H, Ueno T, Sawa Y. Heart transplantation for adults with congenital heart disease: Current status and future prospects. General Thoracic and Cardiovascular Surgery. 2017;**65**:309-320

[6] Koyak Z, Harris L, de Groot JR, et al. Sudden cardiac death in adult congenital heart disease. Circulation. 2012;**126**:1944-1954

[7] Cecchin F, Frangini PA, Brown DW, et al. Cardiac resynchronization therapy (and multisite pacing) in pediatrics and congenital heart disease: Five years experience in a single institution. Journal of Cardiovascular Electrophysiology. 2009;**20**:58-65

[8] Davies RR, Russo MJ, Yang J, Quaegebeur JM, Mosca RS, Chen JM. Listing and transplanting adults with congenital heart disease. Circulation. 2011;**123**:759-767

[9] O'Connor MJ, Lind C, Tang X, et al. Persistence of anti-human leukocyte antibodies in congenital heart disease late after surgery using allografts and whole blood. The journal

of heart and lung transplantation : The official publication of the international society for. Heart Transplantation. 2013;**32**:390-397

[10] Giamberti A, Varrica A, Pome G, et al. The care for adults with congenital heart disease: Organization and function of a grown-up congenital heart disease unit. European Heart Journal Supplements: Journal of the European Society of Cardiology. 2016;**18**: E15-EE8

[11] Bautista-Hernandez V, Thiagarajan RR, Fynn-Thompson F, et al. Preoperative extracorporeal membrane oxygenation as a bridge to cardiac surgery in children with congenital heart disease. The Annals of Thoracic Surgery. 2009;**88**:1306-1311

[12] Belohlavek J, Rohn V, Jansa P, et al. Veno-arterial ECMO in severe acute right ventricular failure with pulmonary obstructive hemodynamic pattern. The Journal of Invasive Cardiology. 2010;**22**:365-369

[13] VanderPluym CJ, Cedars A, Eghtesady P, et al. Outcomes following implantation of mechanical circulatory support in adults with congenital heart disease: An analysis of the interagency registry for mechanically assisted circulatory support (INTERMACS). The Journal of Heart and Lung Transplantation. 2018;**37**:89-99

[14] Krieger EV, Valente AM. Heart failure treatment in adults with congenital heart disease: Where do we stand in 2014? Heart. 2014;**100**:1329-1334

[15] Stout KK, Broberg CS, Book WM, et al. Chronic heart failure in congenital heart disease: A scientific statement from the American Heart Association. Circulation. 2016;**133**: 770-801

[16] Paniagua Martin MJ, Almenar L, Brossa V, et al. Transplantation for complex congenital heart disease in adults: A subanalysis of the Spanish heart transplant registry. Clinical Transplantation. 2012;**26**:755-763

[17] Maly J, Netuka I, Besik J, Dorazilova Z, Pirk J, Szarszoi O. Bridge to transplantation with long-term mechanical assist device in adults after the mustard procedure. The Journal of Heart and Lung Transplantation: The Official Publication of the International Society for Heart Transplantation. 2015;**34**:1177-1181

[18] Everitt MD, Donaldson AE, Stehlik J, et al. Would access to device therapies improve transplant outcomes for adults with congenital heart disease? Analysis of the United Network for Organ Sharing (UNOS). The Journal of Heart and Lung Transplantation: The Official Publication of the International Society for Heart Transplantation. 2011;**30**:395-401

[19] Shah NR, Lam WW, Rodriguez FH, 3rd, et al. Clinical outcomes after ventricular assist device implantation in adults with complex congenital heart disease. The Journal of Heart and Lung Transplantation: The Official Publication of the International Society for Heart Transplantation 2013;**32**:615-620

[20] Newcomb AE, Negri JC, Brizard CP, d'Udekem Y. Successful left ventricular assist device bridge to transplantation after failure of a fontan revision. The Journal of Heart

and Lung Transplantation: The Official Publication of the International Society for Heart Transplantation. 2006;**25**:365-367

[21] Morris CD, Gregoric ID, Cooley DA, Cohn WE, Loyalka P, Frazier OH. Placement of a continuous-flow ventricular assist device in the failing ventricle of an adult patient with complex cyanotic congenital heart disease. The Heart Surgery Forum. 2008;**11**:E143-E144

[22] Stewart AS, Gorman RC, Pocchetino A, Rosengard BR, Acker MA. Left ventricular assist device for right side assistance in patients with transposition. The Annals of Thoracic Surgery. 2002;**74**:912-914

[23] Gelow JM, Song HK, Weiss JB, Mudd JO, Broberg CS. Organ allocation in adults with congenital heart disease listed for heart transplant: Impact of ventricular assist devices. The Journal of Heart and Lung Transplantation: The Official Publication of the International Society for Heart Transplantation. 2013;**32**:1059-1064

[24] Joyce DL, Crow SS, John R, et al. Mechanical circulatory support in patients with heart failure secondary to transposition of the great arteries. The Journal of Heart and Lung Transplantation: The Official Publication of the International Society for Heart Transplantation. 2010;**29**:1302-1305

[25] Maxwell BG, Wong JK, Sheikh AY, Lee PH, Lobato RL. Heart transplantation with or without prior mechanical circulatory support in adults with congenital heart disease. European Journal of Cardio-Thoracic Surgery. 2014;**45**:842-846

[26] Irving C, Parry G, O'Sullivan J, et al. Cardiac transplantation in adults with congenital heart disease. Heart. 2010;**96**:1217-1222

[27] Patel ND, Weiss ES, Allen JG, et al. Heart transplantation for adults with congenital heart disease: Analysis of the united network for organ sharing database. The Annals of Thoracic Surgery 2009;**88**:814-821; discussion 21-2

[28] Taylor DO, Edwards LB, Boucek MM, Trulock EP, Keck BM, Hertz MI. The registry of the international society for heart and lung transplantation: Twenty-first official adult heart transplant report – 2004. The Journal of Heart and Lung Transplantation: The Official Publication of the International Society for Heart Transplantation. 2004;**23**:796-803

[29] Lamour JM, Addonizio LJ, Galantowicz ME, et al. Outcome after orthotopic cardiac transplantation in adults with congenital heart disease. Circulation. 1999;**100**:II200-II205

[30] Bhama JK, Shulman J, Bermudez CA, et al. Heart transplantation for adults with congenital heart disease: Results in the modern era. The Journal of Heart and Lung Transplantation: The Official Publication of the International Society for Heart Transplantation. 2013;**32**:499-504

[31] Karamlou T, Hirsch J, Welke K, et al. A united network for organ sharing analysis of heart transplantation in adults with congenital heart disease: Outcomes and factors associated with mortality and retransplantation. The Journal of Thoracic and Cardiovascular Surgery. 2010;**140**:161-168

[32] Burchill LJ, Edwards LB, Dipchand AI, Stehlik J, Ross HJ. Impact of adult congenital heart disease on survival and mortality after heart transplantation. The Journal of Heart and Lung Transplantation: The Official Publication of the International Society for Heart Transplantation. 2014;**33**:1157-1163

[33] Singh TP, Almond CS, Semigran MJ, Piercey G, Gauvreau K. Risk prediction for early in-hospital mortality following heart transplantation in the United States. Circulation Heart Failure. 2012;**5**:259-266

[34] Karamlou T, Diggs BS, Welke K, et al. Impact of single-ventricle physiology on death after heart transplantation in adults with congenital heart disease. The Annals of Thoracic Surgery. 2012;**94**:1281-1287; discussion 7-8

10

Orthotopic Heart Transplantation: Bicaval Versus Biatrial Surgical Technique

Sofia Martin-Suarez, Marianna Berardi,
Daniela Votano, Antonio Loforte,
Giuseppe Marinelli, Luciano Potena and
Francesco Grigioni

Abstract

In 1967, the first cardiac transplantation was performed in South Africa by Christiaan Barnard, becoming one of the most pioneering events of the human history, comparable to the first step on the moon, 2 years later. Even if Barnard became extremely famous because of this outstanding operation, behind this event there were years and years of studies, experimentations and hard work done by others, in particular by Lower and Shumway. The initial technique, still called 'standard technique' is the biatrial one. In the late 1980s, alternatives like the 'bicaval technique' were developed in order to get a more anatomical result. In the present chapter, we will throw the reader into the early years of the cardiac transplantation era, describing all the efforts made by the "fathers" of the cardiac surgery in order to standardize techniques inherited by the modern surgeons. Afterwards, we will present a review of the literature to answer the question if the biatrial technique should still be called "standard technique".

Keywords: Yacoub, Shumway, tricuspid regurgitation, technical issues

1. Historic background of cardiac transplantation surgical techniques

On December 3, 1967 in Cape Town, Christiaan Barnard performed the first human heart transplant. This was one of the most significant accomplishments in history, allowing to save the life of several patients with end-stage heart disease in the last 50 years. This remarkable surgical innovation was the result of constant work, diligent research, creativity and innovative perception. During the early 1900s, Alexis Carrel, the father of vascular and transplant surgery who was awarded the Nobel Prize in Physiology or Medicine in 1912, and Charles Guthrie, professor of Physiology and Pharmacology at Washington University, performed the first heterotopic heart transplant [1]. Subsequently, other American surgeons, including Mann [2] at Mayo Clinic in 1933 and Marcus [3] at Chicago Medical School two decades later, pursued the experimentation and proposed new techniques for heterotopic heart transplantation. At the same time, on the other side of the world, Vladimir Demikhov at M.V. Lomonosov Moscow State University gave a considerable contribution to this experimental specialty, performing the first combined heart-lung transplant and also the first orthotopic transplant in dogs without the use of hypothermia and pump-oxygenator support. His technique consisted of end-to-side anastomoses between the corresponding thoracic *aortae*, superior *venae cavae*, inferior *venae cavae*, and pulmonary arteries. The donor's inferior pulmonary veins were joined together and connected to the recipient's left atrial appendage. Then, the portion of recipient's heart excluded from circulation was ligated and excised [4]. Unfortunately, Demikhov's research remained unknown for a long time and it was published in English only in 1962.

The introduction of hypothermia and cardiopulmonary bypass in the early 1950s had a decisive impact on heart transplantation research.

In the late 1950s, Shumway and Lower at Stanford University achieved brilliant results experimenting on dogs [5]. They used a simple and effective surgical technique, called "Shumway" or biatrial technique (BA), where the anterior part of donor's left and right atria was incised and anastomosed to the posterior wall of the recipient's atria. This became the standard heart transplant surgical technique until the 1990s. These two pioneers also introduced two innovative methods that allowed to prolong survival times: the use of isotonic saline solution at 4°C to preserve the donor's heart and the use of cardiopulmonary bypass to support the transplanted heart [6].

Based on these promising premises, Shumway begun to think about human heart transplant.

This research recalled the attention of the international scientific community, in particular of Christiaan Barnard, a young South African surgeon with a good reputation in open heart surgery who developed almost an obsession for heart transplantation. In August 1966, he spent 4 months in Lower's laboratory learning the principles of Shumway's research.

At his return to South Africa, on December 3, 1967, he performed the first heart transplant [7]. The donor was Denise Darvall, a 25-year-old woman who had a severe brain injury and was certified brain dead by the neurosurgeons. The recipient was Luois Washkansky, a 53-year-old man with severe heart failure; he died 17 days later due to pneumonia [8].

On December 6, 1967, Adrian Kantrowitz, another pioneer in this field, performed the first pediatric heart transplantation at Maimonides Hospital of New York. The donor was an anencephalic baby and the recipient was an 18-day-old child with Ebstein anomaly. Unfortunately, the young patient died after 6 hours [9].

One month later, on January 6, 1968, Shumway and his team performed the first human heart transplant in the United States. The patient died of gastrointestinal bleeding on the 15th postoperative day.

During the next year, 102 heart transplants were performed around the world, with only 40% survival at 1 year [7]. These poor results were the reason why the most important cardiovascular surgery centers abandoned the procedure.

After these first attempts, heart surgeons realized that specific suppression of the recipient's immune system was required for long-term graft survival. After the introduction of percutaneous transvenous endomyocardial biopsy in 1973, that improved the diagnosis of acute and chronic rejection, and the discovery of cyclosporine A in 1976, a powerful immunosuppressor, better results in terms of survival were achieved, therefore a greater number of procedures was performed [6].

While the "Shumway technique" remained the standard for more than 20 years worldwide, in the early 1990s, some surgeons proposed new effective surgical techniques trying to improve hemodynamic results and late survival [10]. Despite the technical evolution, in the last 50 years, despite the improvement in pharmacological treatment of end-stage heart failure, cardiac transplantation has remained the only treatment (along with left ventricle assistance devices (LVAD) implantation as destination therapy) capable of improving the long-term survival [11, 12]. The standard BA technique, based on the description of Cass and Brock [13] and Lower and Shumway [5] for orthotopic heart transplantation (OHT), was adopted worldwide for many years due to its simplicity and reproducibility. This technique requires, to some extent, the excision of the posterior part of the donor's left atrium and the incision of the right atrium from the inferior vena cava toward the right atrial appendage to avoid injuries to the sino-atrial node. The atrial anastomoses can be performed easily, reducing from 8 possible single-vessel anastomoses for complete transplantation to 4 (**Figure 1**).

However, several studies have demonstrated that the drawback of this technique consists in enlarged, figure-of-eight configured right and left atria without a physiological geometry between the donor and the recipient's atria [14]. This non physiological geometry can lead to (i) higher incidence of mitral and tricuspid valve incompetence, (ii) rhythm disturbances [14] and (iii) tendency of thrombus formation and septal aneurysm [15]. Because of these problems, some authors, as Sir Magdi Yacoub, Banner and Dreyfus some time later [16–18] proposed a more anatomical surgical technique with complete excision of the recipient's atria and direct anastomoses to the left pulmonary veins, right pulmonary veins, inferior venae cavae (IVC), and superior venae cavae (SVC). No technical complications occurred, but the benefit of this procedure on clinical outcome had to be demonstrated, at least in the 1990s.

Sievers and co-workers [19] in 1991, and the Wythenshawe group [20] in 1993, introduced into clinical practice the bicaval transplantation technique (BC), characterized by two arterial, one left atrial, and two caval anastomoses, leaving the right atrium intact and leaving only a small posterior part of recipient's left atrial tissue between the pulmonary veins (**Figure 2**). Potential

Biatrial Technique

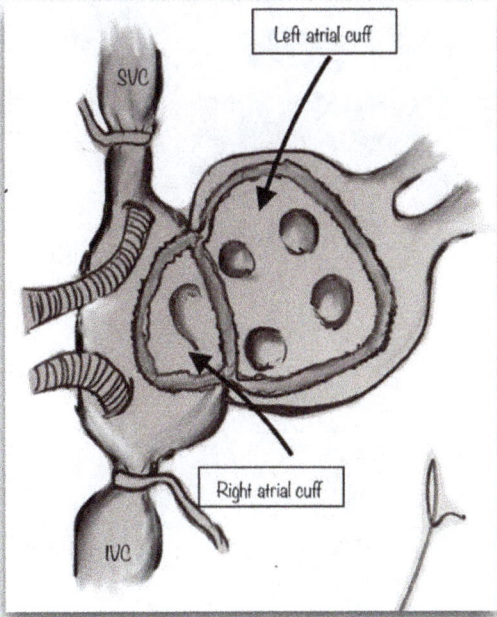

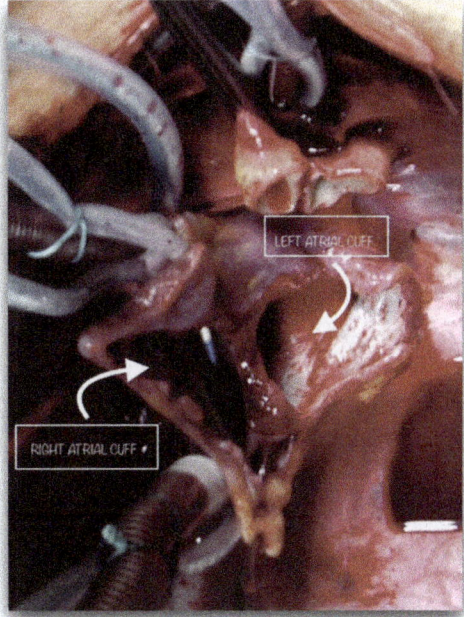

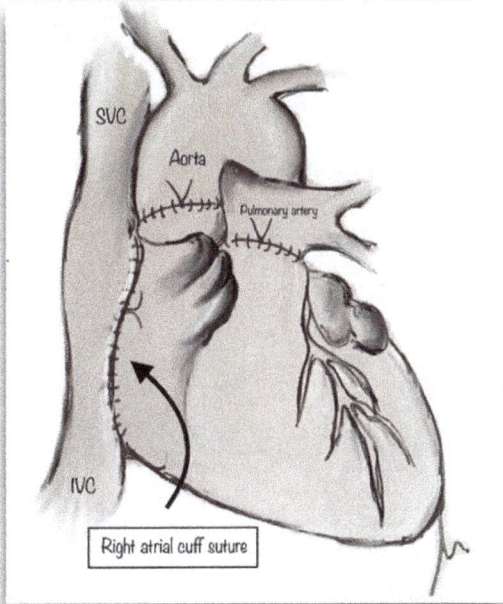

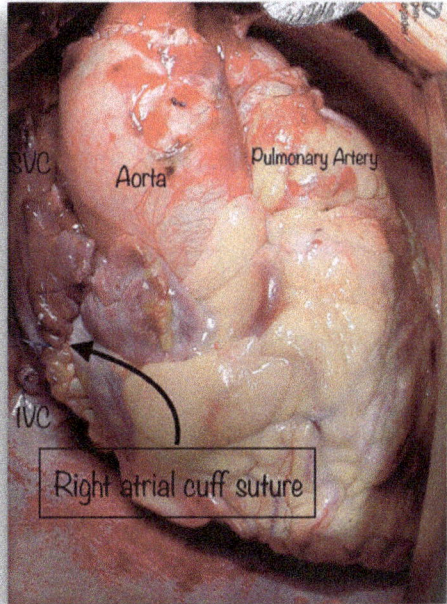

Biatrial Technique

Figure 1. A schema of the Biatrial technique for orthotopic cardiac transplantation is shown. In the left (A), after cardiectomy, the double atrial cuff is distinguishable, with the interatrial septum with the foramen. In the right, (B) the right atrial cuff suture is represented.

Bicaval Technique

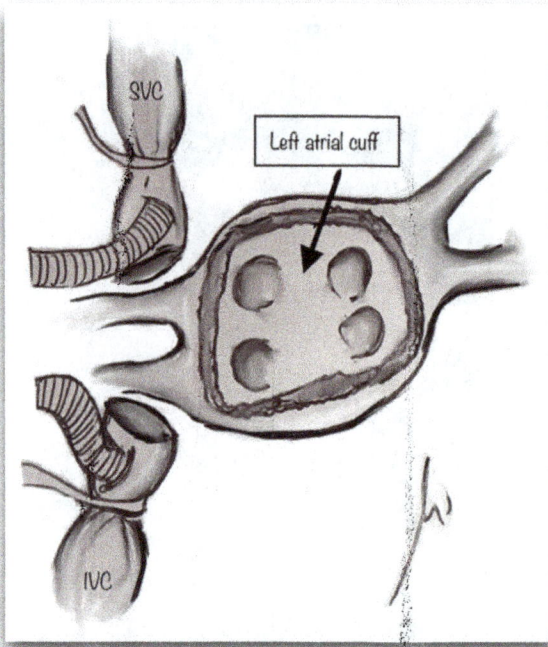

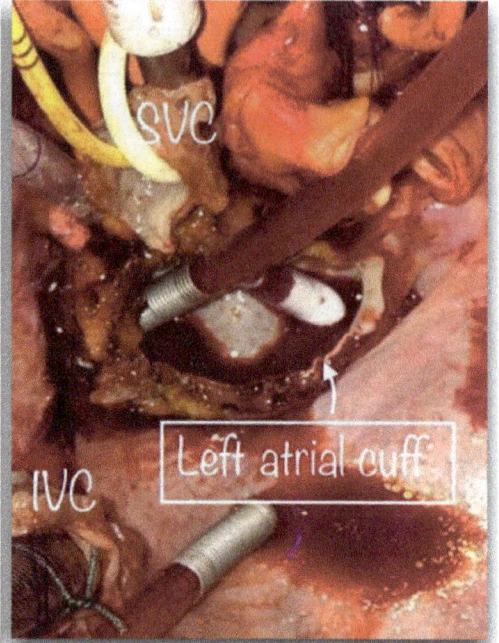

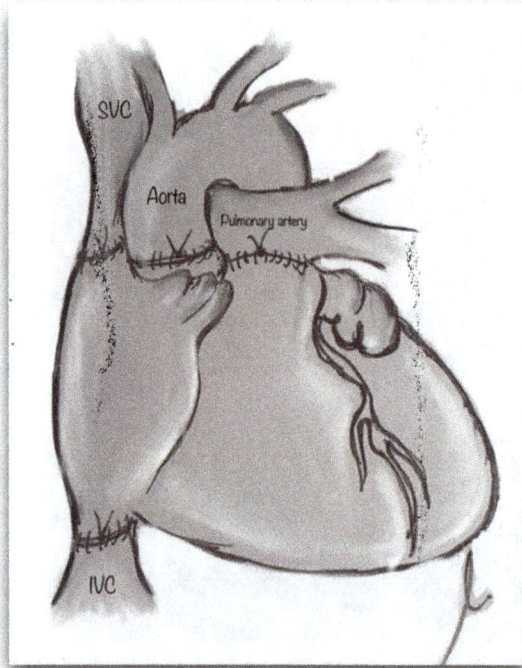

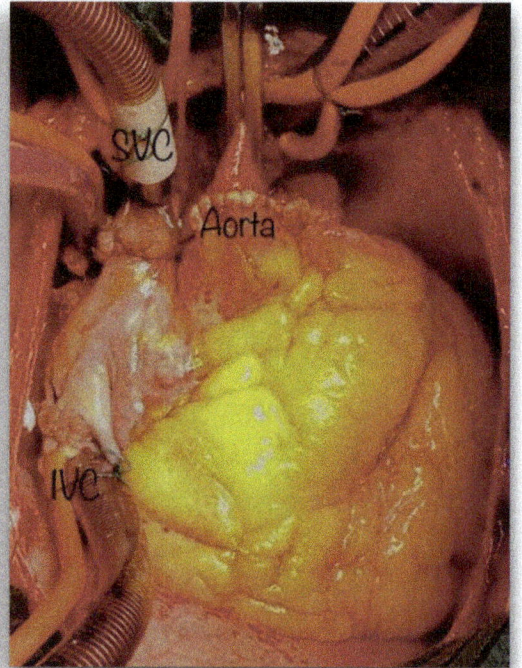

Bicaval Technique

Figure 2. The schema of the Bicaval technique has been designed. In the left side (A), both cavas and the left atrial cuff are prepared after cardiectomy, while in the right side (B) the final result with both superior and inferior vena cava sutures.

shortcomings of the BC technique include the marginally prolonged ischemic transplantation time, which is likely of no clinical relevance, as well as some sort of stenosis at the level of the venous anastomoses. Both problems, however, can be neutralized by refined surgical techniques.

2. Biatrial vs. bicaval technique: Best evidences

During the 1990s, many single center reports, with variable potency and sample size have been published, comparing both techniques from different points of view and outcomes, like post-operative mortality, length of operation in terms of ischemic organ time, length of hospital stay, need for permanent pace maker, echocardiographic findings, exercise capacity and long-term survival.

Remarkable is the paper of Sun et al. [21] with a total of 615 enrolled patients. Among them, 322 were transplanted using the BC technique and 293 using the BA technique. There was no statistically significant difference in terms of early mortality (within 30 post-operative days) between the two groups (3.4% in the BC group vs. 4.8% in the BA group, p 0.5). The average follow-up period was 4.0 ± 3.0 years (ranging from 1 to 11 years). There was no significant difference between groups (3.8 ± 3.5 years in Group 1, 3.8 ± 3.8 years in Group 2). Survival rates at 1, 5 and 10 years were 93, 89 and 87% in the BC group and 89, 82 and 80% in the BA group, respectively. Long-term survival differed significantly between the two groups and the cumulative proportion of survival was significantly higher in the BC group than in the BA group (p 0.05). In the univariate regression analysis, several echocardiographic parameters, such as left atrial diameter, mitral regurgitation, tricuspid regurgitation, left ventricular ejection fraction, right ventricular ejection fraction and surgical techniques, were predictors of long-term survival. Both mitral and tricuspid regurgitation were weakly associated with mortality. There were significant correlations between left and right ventricular ejection fraction and surgical techniques with mortality outcome. Using a multivariate model of analysis, left and right ventricular ejection fraction remained significant risk factors for mortality. When adjusted for left and right ventricular ejection fraction, the surgical techniques (BC vs. BA) significantly influenced mortality outcome in the multivariate analysis. Any significant difference in the incidence of mitral regurgitation between BC and BA transplant patients was demonstrated. However, tricuspid valve regurgitation was much more common in the BA group than in the BC group. They concluded that the BC technique helps to decrease atrial size and tricuspid regurgitation, and better preserves right and left heart function, resulting in improved long-term survival after heart transplantation compared with the BA technique.

Other authors have demonstrated that the BC technique leads to an increased parasympathetic reinnervation compared with the standard technique, which might be of clinical relevance because an increase in blood pressure control, by larger reflex changes in heart rate, might improve adaptation to various stimuli and to physical exercise [22].

However the best way to reach some conclusion is by analyzing papers with the strongest evidences. Relevant among these, two multicenter studies from the UNOS database and other two meta-analysis (see **Table 1**).

Author/ year	Institution	Study Type	Patients	TVR	PM Insertion	Mortality	Survival
Wartig et al. 2014 [30]	Sahlgrenska University Hospital, Gothenburg, Sweden	Retrospective Cohort Study	BA: 221 BC: 226	BA: *Mild*: 103 (37%) *Moderate/ Severe*: 63 (61%)* BC: *Mild*: 169 (61%) *Moderate/ Severe*: 39 (38%)	NA	48 (9.9%)	*1 year*: 84%* *5 years*: 73% *10 years*: 58% *15 years*: 43% *20 years*: 27%
Davies et al. 2010 [23]	Columbia University, New York, USA	Retrospective Review UNOS database	BA: 11.919 (59.3%) BC: 7.661 (38.1%) Total: 519 (2.6%)	NA	BA: 576 (5.1%) BC: 146 (2.0%) Total: 11 (1.9%)	BA: 8.9% BC: 7.6% Total: 9.5%	BA: *1 year*: 85.6%* *5 years*: 72.2%* *10 years*: 51.1%* BC: *1 year*: 87.1% *5 years*: 73.5% *10 years*: 57.4%
Weiss et al. 2008 [24]	Johns Hopkins Medical Institution, Baltimore, USA	Retrospective Review UNOS database	BA: 6.724 BC: 5.207	NA	BA: 343 (5.3%) BC: 103 (2.0%)	BA: *30-days*: 6.6% *1 year*: 13.4% BC: *30-days*: 5.4% *1 year*: 11.5%	BA: *30-days*: 93% *1 year*: 86% *3 years*: 79% *5 years*: 72% BC: *30-days*: 94% *1 year*: 87% *3 years*: 81% *5 years*: 75%
Locali et al. 2008 [28]	Universidade Federal São Paulo, Brazil	Meta-analysis	BA: 914 BC: 872	BA: 310/685 (45.2%) BC: 184/593 (31%)	NA	BA: 102/547 (18.6%) BC: 64/585 (10.9%)	NA
Schnoor et al. 2007 [10]	Medical University Schleswig-Holstein, Luebeck, Germany	Meta-analysis	BA: 1.803 BC: 1.968	BA: 153/261 (58.6%) BC: 61/211 (28.9%)	NA	BA: 18/110 (16.4%) BC: 9/118 (7.6%)	NA

BA: biatrial; BC: bicaval; NA: not analyzed; PM: pace-maker; TVR: tricuspid valve repair; *= p< .01.

Table 1. Overview and outcomes of Biatrial vs. Bicaval for orthotopic heart transplantation.

Davies et al. [23] recently reported from the UNOS data base an analysis of 20,999 transplantations performed on adult patients with no congenital heart disease between 1997 and 2007, including the type of anastomosis performed. Patients were stratified accordingly to the atrial anastomosis technique: standard BA (atrial group, n. 11,919 [59.3%]), BC (caval group, n. 7661 [38.1%]), or total orthotopic (total group, n. 519 [2.6%]). First of all, until 2003, the BA technique was used more frequently than the BC one, while the number of total transplantation decreased. In 2006, more than 34% of the cases of cardiac transplantation were performed with the "standard" or BA technique. The percentage of transplantations performed with the BC technique was higher at higher-volume transplant centers.

Regarding the outcomes, the need for permanent pacemaker was increased in patients in the atrial group (n. 576, 5.1%) requiring a PPM before discharge more often (odds ratio [vs. the caval group], 2.6; 95% CI, 2.2–3.1) than the caval group (n. 146, 2.0%) or the total group (n. 11, 1.9%; odds ratio [vs. the caval group], 1.0, 95% CI, 0.6–1.7). Multivariate predictors of the need for PPM implantation included BA anastomosis (odds ratio, 3.1; 95% CI, 2.5–3.9), donor age of 60–69 years (odds ratio, 2.9; 95% CI, 1.5–5.3), donor age of 50–59 years (odds ratio, 2.0; 95% CI, 1.6–2.5), donor age of 40–49 years (odds ratio, 1.3; 95% CI, 1.0–1.6), recipient inotropic support at transplantation (odds ratio, 1.5; 95% CI, 1.2–1.7), donor history of hypertension (odds ratio, 1.2; 95% CI, 1.0–1.4), and transplantation year (odds ratio, 1.04; 95% CI 1.01–1.07 [per year]); use of T4 before organ retrieval (odds ratio, 0.8; 95% CI, 0.6–0.9) was protective.

In terms of hospital length of stay, patients in the atrial group had longer posttransplantation stay (21.1 days) than those in the caval group (19.3 days, P < 0.0001).

In univariate analysis atrial group patients had a higher incidence of postoperative death (8.9%; odds ratio, 1.17; 95% CI, 1.05–1.30) than those in the caval group (7.6%; odds ratio, 0.83; 95% CI, 0.75–0.93); postoperative mortality in the total group (9.5%; odds ratio, 1.14; 95% CI, 0.86–1.53) was not significantly different from the one seen in either of the other groups. However, the logistic regression model predicting postoperative death did not include the type of anastomosis.

Also in the long-term outcomes, the need for PPM implantation was significantly higher among patients in the atrial group, (P < 0.0001): at 2 years, 8.6% required a pacemaker versus only 5.4% in the BC group and 4.0% in the total group. Multivariate predictors of the interval time between transplantation and PPM insertion included other factors, like recipient age (odds ratio, 1.006; 95% CI, 1.001–1.012 [per year]), transfusions between listing and transplantation (odds ratio, 1.2; 95% CI, 1.0–1.4), donor age of 50 to 59 years (odds ratio, 1.6; 95% CI, 1.3–2.0), donor's age of 60 to 69 years (odds ratio, 2.2; 95% CI, 1.3–3.7), transplantation year (odds ratio, 1.25; 95% CI, 1.21–1.28 [per year]), and BA anastomosis (odds ratio, 2.5; 95% CI, 2.2–2.9); ventricular assistance device at transplantation was protective in this model (odds ratio, 0.7; 95% CI, 0.6–0.9). There was a small but significant difference in long-term survival between the atrial and caval groups in univariate analysis (survival at 1 year, 85.6 vs. 87.1%; at 5 years, 72.2 vs. 73.5%; at 10 years, 51.1 vs. 57.4%; P < 0.0168). Multivariate Cox proportional hazards regression analysis confirmed the decreased survival among patients in the atrial group (hazard ratio, 1.11; 95% CI, 1.04–1.19). There was no difference in graft survival, renal failure-free survival, and transplant coronary atherosclerosis–free survival, based on anastomotic technique.

Three years before the UNOS analysis from Davies et al. [23], Weiss et al. [24] conducted a retrospective review of the UNOS database from January 1999 to December 2005. A total of 14,418 patients underwent first-time OHT during this period. After exclusion of patients aged less than 18 years (n. 1831) and more than 80 years (n. 2), orthotopic total transplants (n. 482), heterotopic transplants (n. 4) and those without data on transplant technique (n. 139), the final study population was 11,931. Of these, 5207 (43%) received the BC anastomotic technique, with follow-up through September 2006. Almost 10,000 patient less than the population analyzed by Davies et al. [23]. Weiss et al. concluded that there was no difference in survival between BC and BA techniques when modeled with long-term follow-up and adjusted for confounding variables. Although the mortality rates were higher for the BA group at 30 days and 1, 3 and 5 years, this represents unadjusted mortality, which disappears in both the logistic regression and proportional hazards model for all time-points. Comparing both studies, we can conclude that probably the results obtained by Davies et al., due to the sample size and the interval period, are complementary to those obtained in the previous Weiss' UNOS analysis, giving more conclusive information. Also the BC technique gives the advantage of decreasing both the need of PPM and the post-operative mortality, but also influences positively the long term survival.

Regarding two relevant meta-analysis, the first one, published by Schnoor et al. [10] in 2007, provides evidences that the expected theoretic advantages of BC transplantation, in comparison with the standard technique, have come true in clinical practice. The meta-analysis included 23 retrospective and 16 prospective studies. In prospective trials, a reduction in right atrial pressure was found. The absolute difference in right atrial pressure is probably of no clinical relevance at rest but it probably could be on exertion. It has been suggested that the patients with BC heart transplant may have superior exercise performance in comparison with BA heart transplant. An attempt to solve this dilemma has been done in 2011 by Czer et al. [25]: he did not found any significant difference in the exercise capacity between patients with BA versus BC techniques for orthotopic heart transplantation. Other factors such as cardiac denervation and immunosuppressive drug effect, or physical deconditioning, may be more important determinants of subnormal exercise capacity after heart transplantation. Nevertheless, the reduction in morbidity and postoperative complications and the simplicity in the BC technique suggest that the BC heart transplantation offers advantages when compared to the standard BA technique.

Another study by Aleksic et al. demonstrated that the BC technique improves resting hemodynamics in patients with high preoperative pulmonary vascular resistance as highlighted by higher cardiac output and index with lower right atrial pressures. Further studies by Aleksic et al. showed that the BC technique improved hemodynamics during episodes of cellular rejection (grade 1B-1R or greater) and during antibody-mediated rejection [26, 27].

Other conclusions from the Schnoor meta-analysis confirmed the outcomes of other single center results, like a higher rate of sinus rhythm after transplantation in the BC group, as well as the significantly reduced rate of tricuspid valve regurgitation, the prevention of contraction abnormalities by the acute atrial enlargement with the standard technique, and the asynchrony of recipient and donor atrial innervation, improving hemodynamic effects after BC transplantation. The enlargement and distension of the atria typical of the standard technique might not only induce an impairment of the electrical impulse initiation and conduction, triggering arrhythmias, but also promote atrial thrombus formation, most likely avoided using the BC technique.

Another relevant meta-analysis is the one conducted by the Brazilian group from San Paolo. Fagionato et al. [28] aimed at increasing the statistical power of the evidences supporting the new techniques against the BA transplantation, thus adding significance to the results of Schnoor et al. They demonstrated many advantages of the BC technique on the BA one: first of all, the ischemia time in the BC group, even when longer, as found in some studies, is compensated by a better cardiac performance with the new techniques, since adequate ventricular filling is dependent on a satisfactory atrial function. Furthermore, the incidence of atrial arrhythmias was lower in the group undergoing BC transplantation, like in Schnoor's study. This can be explained by the preservation of the sino-atrial node integrity. Modifications in the atrial geometry predispose to atrial arrhythmias, as well as increased internal pressure, since these events prolong the electrical conduction time. The severity of the newly developed arrhythmias is known to be also related and proportional to the severity of the rejection. Fagionato's results show no differences between the transplantation techniques in terms of rejection, concluding that the episodes of atrial arrhythmias are mainly due to greater deformity and atrial pressure. In this context, the rejection episodes can also be related to the degree of tricuspid valve regurgitation. In 2002, Aziz et al. [29] showed that individuals with moderate or severe tricuspid regurgitation have a higher number and intensity of rejection events. On the other hand, the progression of cardiac cellular rejection may be accompanied by oedema and papillary muscle dysfunction, or trigger asymmetrical right ventricular contractility, thus leading to tricuspid valve regurgitation. Additionally, the high hydrophilic property of the valve leaflets glycosaminoglycans leads to increased oncotic pressure in the extracellular matrix during cellular rejection, thus causing oedema and precluding adequate function. In this regard, there is another outstanding study conducted from the Swedish group of Wartig et al. [30] that demonstrated in a pretty huge population the impact of the transplantation techniques on the tricuspid function, as well as its impact on survival. Tricuspid valve regurgitation after cardiac transplantation has been argued to be related to the number of biopsies (although this has been found to be contradictory), to the altered geometry of the right atrial anastomosis in the BA technique, to the preoperative recipient's pulmonary vascular resistance, to the ischemic time of the donor's heart, to the donor-recipient size mismatch, to the mismatch between the donor's heart and a large pericardial cavity of the recipient, or to the presence of TR already in the donor. Wartig et al. revised retrospectively their population of transplanted patient since 1984, comparing both cohorts of 221 patients receiving BA technique and 226 receiving BC technique. They observed first that the incidence of early significant TR after HTx was more common after the BA technique than after the BC technique. Furthermore, they demonstrated with a multivariate logistic regression analysis that the BA technique was the only significant predictor of early moderate to severe TR (odds ratio [OR], 2.70; 95% confidence interval [CI], 1.68–4.32; p 0.001). More interestingly, they found that moderate and severe TR at discharge was associated with impaired long-term survival. Moreover, it has been previously shown that the degree of TR is related not only to degree of symptoms and right-sided heart pressures but also to progressive renal dysfunction. When stratifying for technique, we found more patients with significant TR in the BA group at early and also 5-year follow-up, compared to the BC group; however, there was no difference at 10 year of follow-up between groups. The explanation might be that patients in the BA group with significant TR died before 10-year follow-up.

A good option to palliate the high incidence of tricuspid regurgitation is that patients undergoing HTx should have a prophylactic tricuspid valve annuloplasty [31, 32]. This may be a good option using the BA technique is used, but when the BC technique is used, prophylactic tricuspid annuloplasty not only becomes cumbersome intraoperatively, but also unnecessary because none or mild TR appears to be the case in approximately 80% of patients.

In light of these facts, the superiority of the BC technique demonstrated in many scientific relevant papers is undebatable. For this reason, some Authors postulated that the BA transplantation technique should no longer be considered the gold standard for transplantation, and should only be used in selected cases. Thus, today there is no more room for questioning whether there are advantages of the BC or total techniques over the BA technique, but it is legitimate to research possible advantages of one technique over the other, providing the patients with the best treatment.

Author details

Sofia Martin-Suarez[1]*, Marianna Berardi[1], Daniela Votano[1], Antonio Loforte[1], Giuseppe Marinelli[1], Luciano Potena[2] and Francesco Grigioni[2]

*Address all correspondence to: docsofi74@hotmail.com

1 Cardiac Surgery Department, S. Orsola-Malpighi Hospital, Bologna University, Bologna, Italy

2 Cardiology Department, S. Orsola-Malpighi Hospital, Bologna University, Bologna, Italy

References

[1] Carrel A, Guthrie CC. The transplantation of vein and organs. AmMed. 1905;**10**:1101-1102

[2] Mann FC, Priestley JT, Markowitz J, Yater WM. Transplantation of the intact mammalian heart. Archives of Surgery. 1933;**26**:219-224

[3] Marcus E, Wong SN, Luisada AA. Homologous heart grafts: Transplantation of the heart in dogs. Surgical Forum. 1951;**2**:212-217

[4] Cooper DK. Experimental development of cardiac transplantation. British Medical Journal. 1968;**4**:174-181

[5] Lower RR, Shumway NE. Studies on orthotopic homotransplantation of the canine heart. Surgical Forum. 1960;**11**:18-19

[6] DiBardino DJ. The history and development of cardiac transplantation. Texas Heart Institute. 1999;**26**:198-205

[7] Michael LH, Hunt S. Conquering the first hurdles in cardiac transplantation: In the foot-prints of giants. The Journal of Heart and Lung Transplantation. 2017;**36**(12):1276-1278

[8] David KCC. Life's defining moment: Christiaan Barnard and the first human heart trans-plant. The Journal of Heart and Lung Transplantation. 2017;**36**(12):1273-1275

[9] Stolf NAG. History of heart transplantation: A hard and glorious journey. Brazilian Jour-nal of Cardiovascular Surgery. 2017;**32**(5):423-427

[10] Schnoor M, Schafer T, Luhmann D, Sievers HH. Bicaval versus standard technique in orthotopic heart transplantation: A systematic review and meta-analysis. Journal of Tho-racic and Cardiovascular Surgery. 2007;**134**(5):1322-1331

[11] Hamour IM, Khaghani A, Kanagala PK, Mitchell AG, Banner NR. Current outcome of heart transplantation: A 10-year single centre perspective and review. Quarterly Journal of Medicine. 2011;**104**(4):335-43

[12] Slaughter MS, Rogers JG, Milano CA, Russell SD, Conte JV, Feldman D, et al. Advanced heart failure treated with continuous-flow left ventricular assist device. The New England Journal of Medicine. 2009;**361**:2241-2251

[13] Cass MH, Brock R. Heart excision and replacement. Guy's Hospital Reports. 1959;**108**: 285-290

[14] Jacob S, Sellke F. Is bicaval orthotopic heart transplantation superior to the biatrial tech-nique? Interactive Cardiovascular and Thoracic Surgery. 2009;**9**:333-342

[15] Fernandez-Gonzales AL, Llorens R, Herreros JM, et al. Intracardiac thrombi after orthotopic heart transplantation: Clinical significance and etiologic factors. The Journal of Heart and Lung Transplantation. 1994;**13**:236-240

[16] Yacoub M, Mankad P, Ledingham S. Donor procurement and surgical techniques for cardiac transplantation. Seminars in Thoracic and Cardiovascular Surgery. 1990;**2**:153-161

[17] Banner NR, Khaghani A, Fitzgerald M, Mitchell AG, Radley-Smith R, Yacoub MH. The expanding role of cardiac transplantation. In: Unger F, editor. Assisted Circulation. Berlin: Springer-Verlag; 1989

[18] Dreyfus G, Jebara V, Mihaileanu S, Carpentier AF. Total orthotopic heart transplan-tation: An alternative to the standard technique. The Annals of Thoracic Surgery. 1991;**52**: 1181-1184

[19] Sievers HH, Weyand M, Kraatz EG, Bernhard A. An alternative technique for orthotopic cardiac transplantation, with preservation of the normal anatomy of the right atrium. The Thoracic and Cardiovascular Surgeon. 1991;**39**:70-72

[20] Sarsam MA, Campbell CS, Yonan NA, Deiraniya AK, Rahman AN. An alternative surgi-cal technique in orthotopic cardiac transplantation. Journal of Cardiac Surgery. 1993;**8**: 344-349

[21] Sun JP, Niu J, Banbury MK, et al. Influence of different implantation techniques on long-term survival after orthotopic heart transplantation: An echocardiographic study. The Journal of Heart and Lung Transplantation. 2007;**26**:1243-1248

[22] Bernardi L. Influence of type of surgery on the occurrence of parasympathetic reinnervation after cardiac transplantation. Circulation. 1998;**97**:1368-1374

[23] Davies RR, Russo MJ, Morgan JA, et al. Standard versus bicaval techniques for orthotopic heart transplantation: An analysis of the united network for organ sharing database. The Journal of Thoracic and Cardiovascular Surgery. 2010;**140**:700

[24] Weiss ES, Nwakanma LU, Russell SB, Conte JV, Shah AS. Outcomes in bicaval versus biatrial techniques in heart transplantation: An analysis of the UNOS database. The Journal of Heart and Lung Transplantation. 2008;**27**:178-183

[25] Czer LS, Cohen MH, Gallagher SP, Czer LA, Soukiasian HJ, Rafiei M, Pixton JR, Awad M, Trento A. Exercise performance comparison of bicaval and biatrial orthotopic heart transplant recipients. Transplantation Proceedings. 2011;**43**(10):3857-3862

[26] Aleksic I, Freimark D, Blanche C, et al. Does total orthotopic heart transplantation offer improved hemodynamics during cellular rejection events? Transplantation Proceedings. 2003;**35**(1532):2000

[27] Aleksic I, Freimark D, Blanche C, et al. Hemodynamics during humoral rejection events with total versus standard orthotopic heart transplantation. Annals of Thoracic and Cardiovascular Surgery. 2004;**10**:285

[28] Locali RF, Matsuoka PK, Cherbo T, Gabriel EA, Buffolo E. Should biatrial heart transplantation still be performed? A meta-analysis. Arquivos Brasileiros de Cardiologia. 2010;**94**(6):829-840

[29] Aziz TM, Saad RA, Burgess MI, Campbell CS, Yonan NA. Clinical significance of tricuspid valve dysfunction after orthotopic heart transplantation. The Journal of Heart and Lung Transplantation. 2002;**21**(10):1101-1108

[30] Wartig M, Tesan S, Gäbel J, Jeppsson A, Selimovic N, Holmberg E, Dellgren G. Tricuspid regurgitation influences outcome after heart transplantation. The Journal of Heart and Lung Transplantation. 2014;**33**(8):829-835

[31] Fiorelli AI, Oliveira JL, Santos RH, et al. Can tricuspid annuloplasty of the donor heart reduce valve insufficiency following cardiac transplantation with bicaval anastomosis? The Heart Surgery Forum. 2010;**13**:E168-E171

[32] Jeevanandam V, Russell H, Mather P, Furukawa S, Anderson A, Raman J. Donor tricuspid annuloplasty during orthotopic heart transplantation: Long-term results of a prospective controlled study. The Annals of Thoracic Surgery. 2006;**82**:2089-2095

11

Graft Vascular Disease

Lucas Barbieri, Noedir Stolf, Mariane Manso and
Wallace André Pedro da Silva

Abstract

Cardiac transplantation (TxC) is considered the first therapeutic option in patients with congestive heart failure, refractory to clinical treatment and without the possibility of conventional surgical treatment. The pathophysiological status, as a consequence of severe cardiomyopathy, is represented by various degrees of systolic and diastolic dysfunction, reflecting low ejection volumes and high diastolic volumes and high filling diastolic pressures, respectively. Patients in this pathophysiological context also present, among other symptoms, neurohormonal alterations of the renin-angiotensin aldosterone system, decreased renal, visceral and splanchnic perfusion, and increased levels of catecholamines. Barnard et al., in 1967, performed the first orthotopic heart transplantation among humans with relative success, Zerbini (1969) being the first to perform it in Brazil. The presence of high rates of graft rejection and infection accounted for small survival and caused great disinterest and abandonment of the technique in the 70's. However, the experience accumulated by the groups that maintained TxC as a treatment, mainly after the introduction of cyclosporin A, first in kidney transplantation in 1978, and in 1980 in TxC, reinvigorated this therapeutic option, allowing the true development and the application of this treatment worldwide.

Keywords: nanoemulsions, methotrexate, paclitaxel, heart transplantation, allograftvasculopathy

1. Introduction

Cardiac transplantation (TxC) is currently considered the first therapeutic option in patients with congestive heart failure, refractory to clinical treatment and without the possibility of conventional surgical treatment [1].

The pathophysiological status, as a consequence of severe cardiomyopathy, is represented by various degrees of systolic and diastolic dysfunction, reflecting low ejection volumes and high diastolic volumes and high filling diastolic pressures, respectively [2].

Patients in this pathophysiological context also present, among other symptoms, neurohormonal alterations of the renin-angiotensin aldosterone system, decreased renal, visceral, and splanchnic perfusion, and increased levels of catecholamines.

The first reference for heart transplantation is from Carrel and Guthrie, who performed the transplantation of an young animal's heart on the neck of an adult animal [3]. It was, however, the work of Lower and Shumway in the 1950s and 1960s that standardized the technique—which provided a long survival for dogs with immunosuppression—and laid the foundations for the success of this surgical treatment. Barnard et al., in 1967, performed the first orthotopic heart transplantation among humans with relative success, Zerbini being the first to perform it in Brazil [4].

The presence of high rates of graft rejection and infection accounted for small survival and caused great disinterest and abandonment of the technique in the 70's [5, 6]. However, the experience accumulated by the groups that maintained TxC as a treatment, mainly after the introduction of cyclosporin A, first in kidney transplantation in 1978, and in 1980 in TxC, reinvigorated this therapeutic option, allowing the true development and the application of this treatment worldwide.

2. Type of rejection in cardiac transplantation

2.1. Acute cellular rejection

In acute cellular rejection, the antigen-presenting cells directly or indirectly carry the immune message of the graft to the T lymphocyte in a phenomenon known as allorecognition. In this process, the T lymphocyte membrane is bombarded by multiple immune stimuli that activate different effectors, especially calcineurin, which, through interleukin-2, promotes the clonal expansion of T lymphocytes, leading to the production of the following cell clones and enzymes [7, 8].

Auxiliary T lymphocytes (CD4—Helper T lymphocytes) identify antigens on the membrane of cells that have been phagocytosed by macrophages and thereby activate the body's specific immunity;

Cytotoxic T lymphocytes (CD8—Killer T lymphocytes) have the ability to induce lysis of target cells to the case in point the graft cells;

Lymphocytes B are responsible for humoral immunity due to the production of antibodies against foreign antigens, which may give rise to plasma cells (antibody producing cells) or memory cells.

Natural cytotoxic cells (natural killer cells) are granular lymphocytes that destroy target cells by adherence, similar to cytotoxic T lymphocytes (CD8); and the proliferation or rapamycin target enzyme (mTOR—target of rapamycin) regulates the transcription of messenger RNA, acting on growth, proliferation, motility, survival, and protein synthesis of the lymphocyte.

Immunosuppression is generally based on regimens of induction, maintenance, and treatment of acute rejection, described below:

The induction regimen seeks to achieve and induce graft tolerance. This therapy has been reserved for patients at high risk of rejection or renal failure.

- Maintenance therapy usually consists of a therapy combination of corticosteroids, antiproliferative agents, and calcineurin inhibitors. Combination drug therapy seeks to achieve the activation of T cell lymphocytes at various stages, thus allowing lower doses of each drug.

- Rejection or rescue therapy refers to immunosuppressive therapy used to reverse an episode of acute rejection. Rejection is treated by increasing oral therapy with pulses of oral or intravenous corticosteroids with changes in oral therapy or with the use of monoclonal or polyclonal antilymphocytic agents.

2.2. Antibody-mediated rejection

Antibody-mediated rejection can be understood as another form of immune reaction that has a generally more severe course, since circulating preformed antibodies already exists against the alloantigens of the HLA (human leukocyte antigens) graft system. It is a catastrophic situation that leads to acute dysfunction of the organ, and immunosuppressors cannot exert any immediate effect [9–11]. As a preventive measure to curb this event, it has been advocated prior knowledge of the reactivity of the receptor potential to a panel of lymphocytes and the prospective knowledge of cross-lymphocyte testing. In this way, it becomes possible to allocate the donated hearts more rationally to the most suitable recipients.

3. Graft vascular disease

Graft vascular disease in cardiac transplantation is an insidious complication, characterized by persistent perivascular inflammation and intimal hyperplasia. It was first described by Thomson, 1969, and emerges as the most important factor affecting long-term survival after transplantation [12].

Graft vascular disease and coronary atherosclerosis are atheromatous diseases with some similarities and differences in macroscopic and microscopic presentation. Both diseases are characterized by increased cell adhesion and leukocyte infiltration, similar environment and cytokine profiles, aberrant extracellular matrix, and early and prolonged accumulation of extracellular and intracellular lipids, as well as migration of smooth muscle cells, endothelial dysfunction, and abnormality in cellular apoptosis.

It represents a type of rejection in which aggression immune to the coronary endothelium occurs persistently and constitutes the main late complication, limiting the survival of the patient and the graft itself in the long term [13].

Although acute graft failure after transplantation has improved over the last two decades, the same cannot be said in the long run where achievements have been less pronounced. Graft vascular disease appears as the main complication after the first year of transplantation and lacks specific and effective therapy. The importance of this entity can be observed in the comparative analysis of the survival curves presented by the International Society for Heart and Lung Transplantation, in which patients who developed vasculopathy had a higher mortality rate than the others.13 The graft vascular disease is responsible for 17% of the deaths and can be detected as early as the first year after transplantation, reaching in the third year figures in the order of 42% by cinecoronariography and 75% by intravascular ultrasonography [13–17].

The "graft vascular disease" designation has received greater acceptance rather than the other ones—post-transplant atherosclerosis, chronic rejection, accelerated atherosclerosis, graft vasculopathy and others—because it expresses more appropriately the immunological phenomenon that is common to transplants of solid organs [9].

Graft vascular disease is a form of accelerated coronary vasculopathy of immune origin that has not yet been completely clarified, in which nonimmunological factors also take place. However, the most likely entrance door is the endothelial dysfunction, as it allows the aggression of the subintimal layer and stimulates the myointimal proliferation in the wall of the artery. The inflammatory process extends to the entire arterial bed and, occasionally, to the veins, sparing only the recipient's native vessels [8, 18].

In the initial phase of the lesion, there is a discrete thickness of the intima, with little hyperplastic fibrosis and an increase in extracellular matrix proteins. At this stage, the internal elastic lamina is still intact, and the involvement is limited to the proximal arteries. Subsequently, the thickness proceeds diffusely through the coronary vasculature, with the appearance of plaques of fibroadiposal tissue and gradual deposition of calcium with the future formation of isolated plaques of atheroma [19, 20]. The first intimal changes can be observed as early as the sixth month after transplantation [15, 16, 19].

In the late phase of the disease, it is observed that the thickness of the intima is diffuse, with hyperplasia and concentric fibrosis. A detailed study of the coronary arteries has shown the incorporation of lipids and focal plaques of atheromas interspersed with diffuse arteritis [19, 20]. The arteries thickness occurs by the infiltration of mononuclear inflammatory cells in response to alloimmune stimuli or by infection, and in this last situation, the participation of the cytomegalovirus deserves special attention. In a more advanced stage, the medial layer may be totally or partially replaced by fibrous tissue. Only vessels with little or no muscle layer can be spared [21–23].

The participation of acute rejection is controversial in the development of graft vascular disease [24–26]. Among the nonimmunological factors considered to be at risk for graft vascular disease, we highlight those that may compromise the integrity of the endothelium, as classified below [24–29]:

The donor risk factors encephalic death etiology, age, sex, atherosclerotic disease, and his or her clinical characteristics.

As for the receptor: age, sex, cytomegalovirus infection, diabetes mellitus, hypertension, dyslipidemia, smoking, obesity, and hyperhomocysteinemia. Among these are hyperlipidemia and diabetes mellitus with incidence between 50 and 80%.

The first step in triggering graft vascular disease is the recognition that occurs after reperfusion of the graft, aggravated by postanoxic endothelial dysfunction. The major cytokines involved in the rejection process are interleukin-2 (IL-2), interferon-gamma (IFN-γ), and tumor necrosis factor alpha (TNF-α). IL-2 induces proliferation and differentiation of T lymphocytes; IFN-γ activates the macrophages; and TNF-α alone is cytotoxic to the transplanted heart. In addition, TNF-α increases the expression of MHC class I molecules, whereas IFN-γ increases MHC expression of both classes I and II. In general, these cytokines may lead to chronic rejection of the graft. IFN-γ and TNF-α induce the production of vascular cell adhesion molecule 1 (VCAM-1), promoting monocyte adhesion and passage through the endothelium and, consequently, vascular graft disease. Explosive encephalic death promotes greater release of cytokines and adhesion molecules and increases the expression of class I and II antigens of the MHC system, promoting an inflammatory reaction exacerbated in the heart of the potential donor and leading to endothelial dysfunction.

The clinical diagnosis of graft vascular disease is difficult, since myocardial ischemia presents a silent course because it is a denervated heart. In the advanced stage, the disease often manifests with signs of heart failure, arrhythmias or even sudden death [14, 21, 30–32].

Coronary angiography may not express the true severity of the graft vascular disease, since the examination allows only the analysis of the internal diameter of the artery and not of the wall [29, 31–33]. It has been proposed to complement the examination with intravascular ultrasonography, which allows to detect the coronary artery wall thickness even in the initial phase of the process. However, this method is not yet widely used, it is invasive and is limited to analysis only of the largest caliber arteries.

Regarding the noninvasive methods, the dobutamine stress echocardiogram has shown advantages as a non-invasive screening test with good sensitivity to select patients with a higher risk of graft vascular disease [13, 34–36].

Among the alternative surgical methods, direct myocardial revascularization or angioplasty deserves special mention, although both present serious restrictions due to the universal distribution of inflammation in the arteries; therefore, the prognosis of the disease is bleak, and few patients can benefit from retransplantation [31, 37, 38].

Ultimately, effective treatment of graft vascular disease in humans is nonexistent, simply limiting the use of prophylactic measures to reduce risk factors. In this way, the treatment of this terrible disease constitutes a fertile field of research but with multiple challenges.

4. Nanotechnology and nanoscience

Nanotechnology and nanoscience, ranging from 1 to 100 nanometers (nm), focus on materials of atomic size, molecular, and supramolecular, which point to the control and manipulation of these new materials precisely by configuring atoms and molecules, producing new molecular aggregates and designing self-aggregation systems to create supramolecular devices at the cellular or minor scale.

The nanoscale is prevalent in natural systems, as several functional components of living cells fit into this anthropometric classification, but few drugs or diagnostic, therapeutic, and repair devices have been developed on this scale.

The properties of the nanoscale allow high density of function in small packages to minimize invasiveness and facilitate intelligent therapeutic interventions with increased specificity of release and action, decrease of side effects, and ability to respond to external stimuli and to refer to external receptors.

Nanotechnology and nanomedicine are two areas of great growth that have provided new diagnostic and therapeutic opportunities for cardiovascular, pulmonary, hematological, and sleep diseases. In the near future, nanotechnology will play an increasingly significant role in the day-to-day practice of cardiologists, pneumonologists, and hematologists.

The use of nanoparticles in medicine was first performed in the treatment of cancer and progressed rapidly, being well used to address the limitations of conventional drug delivery systems, such as nonspecific and target biodistribution, water solubility, poor oral bioavailability, and low therapeutic indexes.

An effective way to achieve drug delivery efficiency will be to reasonably develop nanosystems based on their knowledge of their interactions with the biological environment, target cell population, changes in cellular receptors that occur with disease progression, mechanism and site of drug action, drug retention, multiple drug administration, molecular mechanism, and pathobiology of the disease under consideration [39].

In the area of biomedical nanotechnology, the group led by Maranhão has made pioneering contributions in the world: they described the first system of nanoparticles (non liposomal) produced in the laboratory, capable of directing and concentrating drugs at the drug targeting site for treatment for the treatment of proliferative diseases such as cancer and atherosclerosis [21, 40, 41] (**Pictures 1** and **2**).

A fascinating field of impact applications has been opened with the discovery that LDE, after injection into the circulatory system, is concentrated in the tumor tissues and can be used in the treatment of cancer as a vehicle to direct chemotherapeutics to the neoplastic cells [42]. The cell probably due to the need for greater lipid content required by accelerated proliferation has a marked increase in the expression of LDL receptors. This enables the use of LDE as a vehicle to concentrate neoplastic neoplastic tissue associated with the particles. Chemotherapeutics are thus diverted from the normal tissues of the organism. Thus, it is possible to increase the therapeutic efficacy of these agents and to reduce the side effects that constitute an important limitation to chemotherapy. The initial finding was described in patients with acute myelocytic leukemia, [40, 41] in whom overexpression of receptors reached up to 100-fold. More recently, it has been found that LDE can also be concentrated in tissues where there are nonneoplastic proliferative processes [43]. Then, in rabbits with

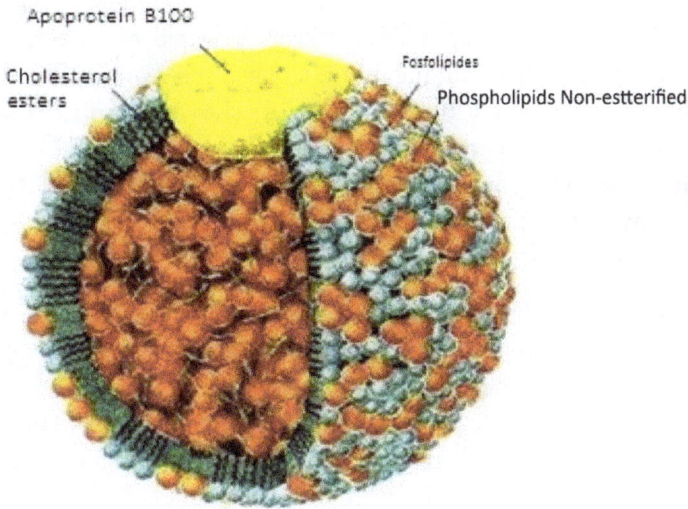

Picture 1. Structure of low density lipoprotein (LDL). Modified from www.foodspace.wordpress.com

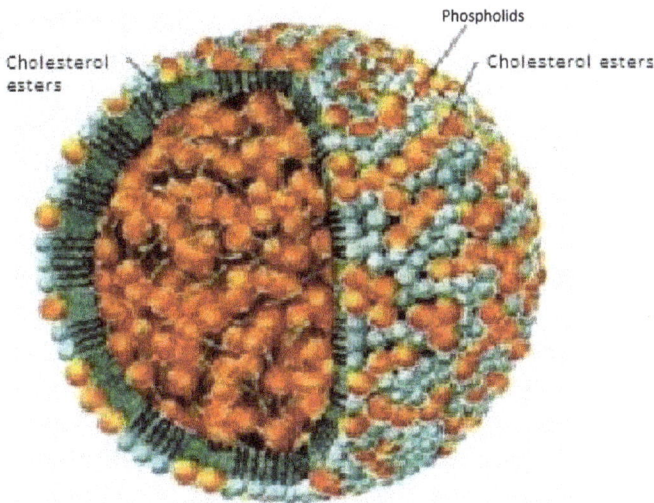

Picture 2. Structure of lipid nanoemulsion (LDE). Modified from www.foodspace.wordpress.com

cholesterol-induced diet atherosclerosis, the inflammatory process in atherosclerosis also led to the concentration of nanoemulsion in injured arteries. These findings broadened the range of potential applications of nanoemulsion as a drug vehicle not only in neoplasias but also in atherosclerosis and other chronic inflammatory processes.

The incorporation and stability of drugs within the LDE were optimized with drug modification without loss of pharmacological effect. Thus, with the modification of these drugs, it was possible to proceed with the assembly of a therapeutic arsenal associated with nanoemulsions.

LDE preparations, associated with modified forms of etoposide chemotherapeutic agents, paclitaxel 18 and methotrexate, are ready and efficiently tested in vitro and in vivo. In all cases, comparing these associations with nanoemulsions to the respective commercial preparations, a greater therapeutic action at higher doses was shown in culture of neoplastic cells and models of tumors implanted in animals (Walker's tumor and B-16 melanoma). In clinical trials with carmustine, etoposide, and paclitaxel [18, 20, 42], it was found that in the use of these drugs associated with LDE, even at higher doses than those usually used in the clinic, the toxicity was practically absent.

The results described above then directed us to the application of these nanoemulsions in the treatment of patients with heart transplantation, in which two main problems predominate: rejection of the receptor to the transplanted organ and the SVD. These are two entities that are difficult to manage clinically, which seriously compromise the success of heart transplants and which require new therapeutic solutions. For DVE, in general, there is no conventional treatment, only retransplantation. The inflammatory and proliferative bases of SVD are similar to those of atherosclerotic cardiovascular disease. Thus, the fact that an antiproliferative agent associated with LDE has been effective in promoting the regression of experimental atherosclerosis suggests that it is equally efficient as a therapeutic approach to PVD.

Author details

Lucas Barbieri[1]*, Noedir Stolf[1], Mariane Manso[2] and Wallace André Pedro da Silva[3]

*Address all correspondence to: lucasbarbieri@usp.br

1 FMUSP-Incor, hospital BP, São Paulo, Brasil

2 FMABC, Santo André, São Paulo, Brasil

3 Hospital Geral de Palmas, Palmas, Brasil

References

[1] Korewicki J. Cardiac transplantation is still the method of choice in the treatment of patients with severe heart failure. Cardiology Journal. 2009;16(6):493-499

[2] Ramakrishna H, Jaroszewski DE, Arabia FA. Adult cardiac transplantation: A review of perioperative management part-I. Annals of Cardiac Anaesthesia. 2009;12(1):71-78

[3] Silva PR. Transplante cardíaco e cardiopulmonar: 100 anos de história e 40 de existência. Revista Brasileira de Cirurgia Cardiovascular. 2008;23(1):145-152

[4] Fiorelli AI, Coelho HB, Oliveira Junior JL, Oliveira AS. Insuficiência cardíaca e transplante cardíaco. Rev. Med. (São Paulo). 2008;87(2):105-120

[5]   Griepp RB, Stinson EB, Clark DA, Shumway NE. A two-year experience with human heart transplantation. California Medicine. 1970;**113**(2):17-26

[6]   Rider AK, Copeland JG, Hunt SA, Mason J, Specter MJ, Winkle RA, et al. The status of cardiac transplantation. Circulation. 1975;**52**(4):531-539

[7]   Miller LW, Granville DJ, Narula J, Mcmanus BM. Apoptosis in cardiac transplant rejection. Cardiology Clinics. 2001;**19**:141-154

[8]   Rogers NJ, Lechler RI. Allorecognition. American Journal of Transplantation. 2001;**1**:97-102

[9]   Jukes JP, Jones ND. Immunology in the clinic review series; focus on host responses: Invariant natural killer T cell activation following transplantation. Clinical and Experimental Immunology. 2012;**167**:32-39

[10] Weis M, Von Scheidt W. Coronary artery disease in the transplanted heart. Annual Review of Medicine. 2000;**5**(1):81-100

[11] Diujvestijn AM, Derhaag JG, Van Breda Vriesman PJ. Complement activation by anti-endothelial cell antibodies in MHC-mismatched and MHC-matched heart allograft rejection: Anti-MHC-but not anti non-MHC alloantibodies are effective in complement activation. Transplant International. 2000;**13**:363-371

[12] Lourenço-Filho DD, Maranhão RC, Méndez-Contreras CA, Tavares ER, Freitas FR, Stolf NA. An artificial nanoemulsion carrying paclitaxel decreases the transplant heart vascular disease: A study in a rabbit graft mod el. The Journal of Thoracic and Cardiovascular Surgery. 2011;**141**:1522-1528

[13] Rora P, Edwards LB, Kucheryavaya AY, Christie JD, Dobbels F, Kirk R, et al. The registry of the International Society for Heart and Lung Transplantation: Thirteenth official pediatric lung and heart-lung transplantation report—2010. The Journal of Heart and Lung Transplantation. 2010;**29**:1129-1141

[14] Fiorelli AI. Contribuição ao estudo da função do ventrículo esquerdo no pós-operatório de transplante cardíaco. Tese (Doutorado). São Paulo: Faculdade de Medicina da Universidade de São Paulo; 1992

[15] Fiorelli AI, Stolf NAG, Graziosi P, Bocchi EA, Busnardo F, Gaiotto FA, et al. Incidência de coronariopatia após o transplante cardíaco ortotópico. Revista Brasileira de Cirurgia Cardiovascular. 1994;**9**:69-80

[16] Bacal F, Veiga VC, Fiorelli AI, Bellotti G, Bocchi EA, Stolf NA, et al. Analysis of the risk factors for allograft vasculopathy in asymptomatic patients after cardiac transplantation. Arquivos Brasileiros de Cardiologia. 2000;**75**:421-428

[17] Kobashigawa JA, Tobis JM, Starling RC, Tuzcu EM, Smith AL, Valantine HA, et al. Multicenter intravascular ultrasound validation study among heart transplant recipients: Outcomes after five years. Journal of the American College of Cardiology. 2005;**45**:1532-1537

[18] Van Loosdregt J, Van Oosterhout MF, Bruggink AH, Van Wichen DF, Van Kuik J, De Koning E, et al. The chemokine and chemokine receptor profile of infiltrating cells

in the wall of arteries with cardiac allograft vasculopathy is indicative of a memory T-helper 1 response. Circulation. 2006;**114**:1599-1607

[19] Weis M, Von Scheidt W. Coronary artery disease in the transplanted heart. Annual Review of Medicine. 2000;**51**:81-100

[20] Labarrere CA, Nelson DR, Faulk WP. Myocardial fibrin deposits in first month after transplantation predict subsequent coronary artery disease and graft failure in cardiac allograft recipients. The American Journal of Medicine. 1998;**105**:207-213

[21] Aranda JM, Hill J. Cardiac transplant vasculopathy. Chest. 2000;**118**:1792-1800

[22] Wehner J, Morrell CN, Reynolds T, Rodriguez ER, Baldwin WM III. Antibody and complement in transplant vasculopathy. Circulation Research. 2007;**100**:191-203

[23] Billingham ME. Histopathology of graft coronary disease. The Journal of Heart and Lung Transplantation. 1992;**11**:S38-S44

[24] Costanzo-Nordin MR. Cardiac allograft vasculopathy: Relationship with acute cellular rejection and histocompatibility. The Journal of Heart and Lung Transplantation. 1992; **11**:S90-S103

[25] Hammond EH, Yowell RL, Nunoda S, Menlove RL, Renlund DG, Bristow MR, et al. Vascular (humoral) rejection in heart transplantation: Pathologic observations and clinical implications. The Journal of Heart Transplantation. 1989;**8**:430-443

[26] Kemna MS, Valantine HA, Hunt SA. Metabolic risk factors for atherosclerosis in heart transplant recipients. American Heart Journal. 1994;**128**:68-72

[27] Colvin-Adams M, Agnihotri A. Cardiac allograft vasculopathy: Current knowledge and future direction. Clinical Transplantation. 2011;**25**:175-184

[28] Sambiase NV, Higuchi ML, Nuovo G, Gutierrez PS, Fiorelli AI, Uip DE, et al. Cmv and transplant-related coronary atherosclerosis: An immunohistochemical, in situ hybridization, and polymerase chain reaction in situ study. Modern Pathology. 2000;**13**:173-179

[29] Schmauss D, Weis M. Cardiac allograft vasculopathy: Recent developments. Circulation. 2008;**117**:2131-2141

[30] Rahmani M, Cruz RP, Granville DJ, McManus B. Allograft vasculopathy versus atherosclerosis. Circulation Research. 2006;**99**(8):801-815

[31] Crespo-Leiro MG, Marzoa-Rivas R, Barge-Caballero E,Paniagua-Martín MJ. Prevention and treatment of coronary artery vasculopathy. Current Opinion in Organ Transplantation. 2012;**17**:546-550

[32] Costanzo MR, Naftel DC, Pritzker MR, Heilman JK 3rd, Boehmer JP, Brozena SC, et al. Heart transplant coronary artery disease detected by coronary angiography: A multi-institutional study of preoperative donor and recipient risk factors. Cardiac Transplant Research Database. Journal of Heart and Lung Transplantation. 1998;**17**:744-753

[33] Bocchi EA, Higuchi ML, Bellotti G, Kowabota VS, Assis RV, Stolf N, et al. Acute myo-cardial infarction with diffuse endarteritis, contraction bands, and distal thrombosis of the coronary arteries in a heart transplant patient. The Journal of Heart and Lung Transplantation. 1992;**11**:31-36

[34] Sade LE, Sezgin A, Eroglu S, Bozbas H, Uluçam M, Müderrisoglu H. Dobutamine stress echocardiography in the assessment of cardiac allograft vasculopathy in asymptomatic recipients. Transplantation Proceedings. 2008;**40**:267-270

[35] Eroglu E, D'hooge J, Sutherland GR, Marciniak A, Thijs D, Droogne W, et al. Quantitative dobutamine stress echocardiography for the early detection of cardiac allograft vascu-lopathy in heart transplant recipients. Heart. 2008;**94**:e3

[36] Bacal F, Moreira L, Souza G, Rodrigues AC, Fiorelli A, Stolf N, et al. Dobutamine stress echocardiography predicts cardiac events or death in asymptomatic patients long-term after heart transplantation: 4-year prospective evaluation. The Journal of Heart and Lung Transplantation. 2004;(23):1238-1244

[37] Prada-DelgadoO,Estévez-LoureiroR,López-SainzA,Gargallo-FernándezP,Paniagua-MartínMJ, Marzoa-Rivas R, et al. Percutaneous coronary interventions and bypass surgery in patients with cardiac allograft vasculopathy: A single-center experience. Transplantation Proceedings. 2012;**44**:2657-2659

[38] Bocchi EA, Vilas-Boas F, Pedrosa AA, Bacal F, Fiorelli A, Ariê S, et al. Percutaneous trans-luminal coronary angioplasty after orthotopic heart transplantation. Arquivos Brasileiros de Cardiologia. 1994;**62**:177-179

[39] Suri SS, Fenniri H, Singh B. Nanotechnology-based drug delivery systems. Journal of Occupational Medicine and Toxicology. 2007;**2**:16

[40] Maranhão RC, Garicochea B, Silva EL, Dorlhiac-Llacer P, Pileggi FJC, Chamone DAF. Increased plasma removal of microemulsions resembling the lipid phase of low-density lipoproteins (LDL) in patients with acute myeloid leukemia: A possible new strategy for the treatment of the disease. Brazilian Journal of Medical and Biological Research. 1992;**25**:1003-1007

[41] Maranhão RC, Garicochea B, Silva EL, Dorlhiac-Llacer P, Cadena SM, Coelho IJ, et al. Plasma kinetics and biodistribution of a lipid emulsion resembling low density lipopro-tein in patients with acute leukemia. Cancer Research. 1994;**54**:4660-4666

[42] Maranhão RC, Graziani SR, Yamaguchi N, Melo RF, Latrilha MC, Rodrigues DG, et al. Association of carmustine with a lipid emulsion: In vitro, in vivo and preliminary stud-ies in cancer patients. Cancer Chemotherapy and Pharmacology. 2002;**49**:487-498

[43] Naoum FA, Gualandro SF, Latrilha MC, Maranhão RC. Plasma kinetics of a cholesterol-rich microemulsion in subjects with heterozygous Beta-thalassemia. American Journal of Hematology. 2004;**77**(4):340-345

12

Anesthesia and Intensive Care Management for Cardiac Transplantation

Massimo Baiocchi, Maria Benedetto,
Marta Agulli and Guido Frascaroli

Abstract

Patient management in heart transplant is quite complex and includes multiple steps from preoperative recipient evaluation to postoperative ICU treatment. Monitoring, anesthesia induction, and cardiopulmonary bypass weaning strategies are discussed. The success of the operation also depends on right heart support especially in case of pulmonary hypertension. Many details like fluid management, well-timed respiratory weaning, and primary graft dysfunction management can make the difference in terms of outcome. Pediatric heart transplants represent a small group of total cardiac transplant, but the differences in anatomy and physiology make the surgical and anesthesiological management more complex in unique scenario that requires a specific knowledge at different stages of growth, from newborn through childhood up to adulthood.

Keywords: anesthesia, intensive care, monitoring, inotropic drugs, mechanical support

1. Intraoperative management

Intraoperative management in heart transplant is quite complex and includes multiple steps from preoperative evaluation to ICU admission.

1.1. Preoperative evaluation

During this phase, we need to collect the consent from the patient after having explained to him all the possible complications coming from surgery, anesthesia, and ICU stay.

Above all, we need to know the background history of the patient, any previous issue with general anesthesia, allergies, difficult airway management, and any possible contraindication to the transplant itself [**Table 1**].

A multiorgan analysis must be taken into account:

- Neurological history: syncopal episodes, carotid stenosis, ischemic or hemorrhagic stroke, transitory ischemic attack.

- Respiratory history: smoke, COPD, spirometry, DLCO test.

- Cardiovascular history:

  1. origin of cardiomyopathy: dilated/hypertrophic/ischemic cardiomyopathy

  2. noncompaction left ventricle (LV), sarcoidosis, amyloidosis, and others

  3. arrhythmias: episodes of sudden cardiac death syndrome, implantation of an ICD

  4. right side catheterization: pulmonary artery pressures (PAP), pulmonary capillary wedge pressure (PCWP), pulmonary vascular resistances (PVR), results of reversibility test with enoximone, origin of pulmonary hypertension (prepost capillary)

  5. presence of prosthetic valves in situ

  6. home medications: oral anticoagulants, ace inhibitors, b-blockers, diuretics

- Renal history: chronic or acute renal failure, preoperative serum level of creatinine and urea, creatinine clearance, history of renal replacement therapy.

- Hepatobiliary history: a systemic portal venous congestion can often derive from chronic congestive heart failure. In this case, high levels of transaminases and bilirubin may occur and this may influence the pharmacological and hemodynamic management during anesthesia.

Absolute contraindications	Relative contraindications
Significant COPD (FEV1 < 1 L/min)	Age > 72 years
Fixed pulmonary hypertension	Active infections
PAPs >60 mmHg	BMI > 35 kg/m^2 or <18 kg/m^2
GTP > 15 mmHg	Creatinine clearance < 25 ml/min
PVR > 6 wood units	Active mental illness or psychosocial instability
Irreversible renal or hepatic dysfunction	Severe peripheral vascular disease
AIDS/malignancy/lupus	Diabetes mellitus with end organ damage

Table 1. Contraindications to heart transplantation.

- Metabolic history: surgical stress and corticosteroid therapy may dramatically increase glycemia levels and hyperglycemia may dramatically increase the lactate levels during and after surgery; this is the reason why we need to know if the patient has diabetes and plan a proper blood glucose control with continuous infusion insulin (usually 50 UI/50 ml gelatin starting with a speed of 2–3 ml/h, depending on glucose plasma levels, with a target of 80–150 mg/dl). Among metabolic disorders, hypothyroidism can be further impaired during and after heart transplantation because plasma levels of triiodothyronine are often decreased during long periods of cardiopulmonary bypass, so that it's important to plan an early replacement thyroid therapy.

- Preoperative fasting: the patient should fast from food at least 8 hours and from fluids 4–6 hours before the operation.

- Premedication: it's important to avoid any preoperative oversedation since hypoxia may increase the pulmonary vascular resistances (PVR). We usually do not exceed a dose of $10-15$ drops per os of diazepam in adult patients before going to theater, but, if the patient is really critical, we avoid any premedication.

1.2. Recipient with pulmonary hypertension

Severe pulmonary hypertension in the recipient is one of the major contraindications to heart transplant [1, 2] due to high risk of right heart failure. When pulmonary hypertension persists up to 1 year from transplant, clinical outcomes and percentage of long-term survival are really poor [3]. For the above-mentioned reasons, a potential recipient must be evaluated with caution before being added to the waiting list. First of all, he needs to be sent for cath lab in order to evaluate his own pulmonary vascular resistances (PVR), mean pulmonary arterial pressure (m-PAP), pulmonary artery wedge pressure (PAWP), cardiac output (CO), cardiac index (CI), and the transpulmonary gradient (TPG).

This last equals the difference between mPAP and wedge pressure (TPG = mPAP − PAWP).

In case of high PVR (PVR > 3 wood units [WU]), it is important to perform the reversibility test with enoximone or dobutamine in order to quantify the reversibility degree of pulmonary hypertension. When postcapillary pulmonary hypertension (defined as mPAP $\geq$ 25 mmHg, PAWP > 15 mmHg and PVR > 3WU) is unresponsive to dobutamine reversibility test (i.e., PVR > 3 WU or mPAP > 35 mmHg with a TPG > 12 mmHg), a team made of cardiologists, anesthesiologists, and cardiac surgeons should seriously evaluate if the patient is suitable for receiving a new heart.

A preventive treatment with pulmonary vasodilators such as sildenafil should be considered since it has been shown to decrease the PVR in a period of few months [4].

A preventive treatment with sildenafil should also be considered when patients are scheduled for receiving an LVAD positioning as bridge to transplant, thanks to its effectiveness in long-term reduction of the PVR and major responsiveness to a further test with dobutamine [5].

2. Monitoring and induction of general anesthesia

Timing to get the patient ready to receive the new organ is crucial because the ischemia of the donor heart should be as short as possible to avoid the ischemia-reperfusion injury.

Everyone in the theater should wear sterile surgical gown, hat, mask, and sterile gloves for any procedure on the patient especially because he will go under immune deficiency. Once the patient is in the theater, he will be connected to multiparametric monitor, with the 12 lead ECG and oximetry probe. Two peripheral venous lines are placed (generally 18G for iv sedation and 14G for rapid fluid infusion), and an arterial catheter, generally 20G, is placed into the radial or humeral artery. When the patient is very unstable, an arterial catheter is placed in the left femoral artery, to estimate central to peripheral arterial pressure gradients. Placement of an arterial line can be very difficult in patients with previous implantation of LVADs as bridge to transplant, due to the absence of arterial pulse. In such situations, ultrasound guidance can be very helpful (see **Table 2**).

Induction of general anesthesia usually starts just with the final acceptance of the donor organ. Drugs used for general anesthesia should impact the less possible on hemodynamics. A rapid sequence induction is preferred since recipients are always very stressed and sometimes not present with an empty stomach [6].

Midazolam (10–15 mg) or etomidate (20 mg) are preferred to propofol for hypnosis, due to the less impact on hemodynamics. Opioids like fentanyl or sufentanil are preferred for the same reason ("stress-free anesthesia"), with an induction dose of 0.2–0.4 mcg/kg for sufentanil and 2–4 mcg/kg for fentanyl. Continuous infusion analgesia remifentanil is preferable for the less impact on renal function since it is metabolized by plasmatic esterase. This is particularly important in patients with low cardiac output and preexisting renal failure. Remifentanil will be turned off and replaced by morphine or tramadol (30 mg/die and 300 mg/die, respectively), before moving to the intensive care unit. Mean term muscle relaxant rocuronium (1 mg/kg) is usually the first choice for rapid sequence induction. Sometimes short-term cisatracurium

Device	Measure
PA radial	Invasive arterial pressure (peripheral)
PA fem	Invasive arterial pressure (central)
CVP	Central venous pressure
ECG	12 lead electrocardiography
SpO2	Oxygen saturation levels
PAC	(pulmonary artery catheter) PAPs, PAPm, PAPd, sVO_2
TEE	Biventricular function, shape of ventricular septum, filling, air etc.
NIRS	$ScvO_2$ correlation, adequate tissue perfusion, brain perfusion
LAP	LV filling pressure

Table 2. Standard monitoring.

besylate (0.15–0.2 mg/kg for induction and 1–2 mcg/kg/min for continuous iv infusion during surgery) is a good alternative since it is metabolized by ester hydrolysis and Hofmann reaction, so the duration of block is not affected by renal or hepatic function. During induction of general anesthesia, severe hypotension can occur, so that a fluid iv bolus ad availability of rapid onset vasoconstrictors as metaraminol, phenylephrine, noradrenaline should be ensured. Cardioplegia is not administered in the recipient during heart transplantation, so that the risk of related hemodilution is less than routine cardiac surgery. On pump, sevoflurane or iv 2% propofol infusion (4 mg/kg/h) are the options for maintenance of general anesthesia. Monitoring the depth of anesthesia with bispectral index (BIS) should be routinely adopted in order to decrease the risk of awareness. Once having put the patient asleep, central lines must be placed (queen central venous pressure [CVP] line and 8 Fr line for the pulmonary artery catheter [PAC]). The ideal site for puncture (blind or ultrasound-guided) is the left internal jugular vein (IJV), since the right one can be reserved for eventual postoperative biopsy (necessary to evaluate the level of graft rejection). When this is not possible (presence of ICD on the left side), we can adopt the right subclavian vein. Sometimes, when the preoperative renal function is really compromised, we can already place into the femoral or subclavian vein a catheter for continuous renal filtration afterwards. The PA catheter is flown through the 8 Fr line up to the right atrium, and then, once the new heart is placed, it will be advanced by the cardiac surgeon up to the superior right pulmonary artery. Vigilance calibration will be done immediately before weaning from the CPB.

3. CPB and weaning

If the graft is not carried out into the organ care system (OCS), the ischemic time is crucial and the risk of ischemic/reperfusion injury is proportionally high, with possible dramatic increase of blood lactate levels and decrease of the graft global function. This is the reason why we must ensure adequate glycemia control, urine output, and, in general, an optimal tissue perfusion during CPB. This means to guarantee an adequate oxygen delivery (DO_2), which means to keep MAPs about 60–80 mmHg and Hb levels at least about 8–9 mg/dL. When the aorta is unclamped, VF can occur (50% of patients). A shock delivery (10–30 J) followed by lidocaine bolus (when VF is refractory to electrical therapy) will take to resolution of the arrhythmia and return to sinus rhythm. In case of sinus bradycardia, temporary epicardial pacing will ensure adequate heart rate (100–110 bpm). Due to limited muscular mass, the ability of the right ventricle (RV) to increase contractility is limited and a temporary pacing at about 110 bpm will increase RV output and will overpace possible arrhythmias. Surgeons will also place a left atrial catheter for continuous measurement of the left atrial pressure (LAP) as an indicator of the left ventricle performance and stiffness. This value, together with CVP, PAPs, MAPs, and SvO2, will influence the posttransplantation hemodynamic management. Throughout this period, it will be mandatory to ensure adequate MAPs and diastolic pressure to allow adequate coronary perfusion, while maintaining medium-low preload pressures (CVP < 12 mmHg, LAP/PCWP < 12 mmHg). The biventricular assessment with transesophageal echocardiography should be done simultaneously.

Pharmacological tools for CPB weaning will include the following [**Tables 3** and **4**]:

- Isoprenaline at low-moderate dose (0.02–0.04 mcg/kg/min): it is the first choice in heart transplantation due to the positive chronotropic effect; it helps to guarantee a heart rate of 100–110 bpm. If it does not work, do not go beyond 0.04 mcg/kg/min, in order to avoid hypotensive effects. In this case, switching to atrial pacing is the best choice.

- Adrenaline (0.02–0.2 mcg/kg/min): it provides inotropic support to the new heart, especially to the right ventricle, which is the one more at risk of failure.

- Milrinone (0.2–0.5 mcg/kg/min) or other phosphodiesterase inhibitors (enoximone at 5–8 mcg/kg/min): they increase contractility especially of the right ventricle, while decreasing pulmonary vascular resistances. They both increase intracellular levels of cAMP, but they also decrease the systemic vascular resistances (SVR), so that the patient may benefit from low-moderate noradrenergic support in addition. If systemic peripheral resistances are really low, selective pulmonary vasodilators, aimed to decrease RV afterload without affecting peripheral resistances, are a better choice: inhaled nitric oxide (iNO) at 20–40 ppm [9, 17]) or aerosolized prostaglandins (iloprost 20 mcg/15 min, repeated after 4 hours).

  Possible side effects of these selective inhalation drugs are inhibition of platelet activation and aggregation and inhibition of leucocyte adhesion.

- Levosimendan (0.1–0.2 mcg/kg/min) has also been reported to reverse low cardiac output after heart transplantation [10], although its use has not been shown to reduce cardiac surgery mortality [11].

After having unclamped the aorta and before weaning from CPB, about 1 hour of assistance to the new heart is provided. During this period, an adequate temperature is achieved (36–36.5°C measured by nasopharyngeal temperature probe). Vigilance calibration is performed by providing Hb levels and SvO_2 from gas analysis; it gives results about the indexed cardiac output, pulmonary vascular resistances, and systemic peripheral vascular resistances, indexed on the patient weight. PAPs are shown on the monitor together with CVP, LAP, MAPs, and ECG. The PAVR (pulmonary artery vascular resistance) equals: PAVR = [80 × (mean pulmonary artery pressure – pulmonary + capillary wedge pressure)/cardiac output] (normal value 100 dynes/cm^{-5}).

The TPG (transpulmonary gradient) equals: TPG = mPAP – PCWP (normal value 6 mmHg).

A TPG > 15 mmHg is considered at high risk to develop early postoperative RV dysfunction [7]. The reason for RV dysfunction development may be found in the background of the donor heart. Especially when young and comparably small, it may not easily adapt to the already existing pulmonary hypertension in the recipient. Furthermore, as a result of a long ischemia and CPB time, with ischemia-reperfusion injury, RV dilates, becomes ischemic, and further reduces its own contractility. In this case, we need to adjust the amount of inotropes, chronotropes, and pulmonary vasodilators given, basing also on transesophageal echocardiography that can show the biventricular systolic-diastolic function and fluid responsiveness. Once the patient is stable and the heart rate is appropriate, we can start ventilation and slowly decrease the pump flow until 0.5–1 L/min. At that point, we come out from bypass. During CPB weaning, the heart should be loaded with caution because RV is very sensitive to distension. Echocardiographic parameters to asses the RV behavior will be RVFAC (fractional area change), leftward shift of

Sustain SVR and arterial pressure (if necessary)	Norepinephrine
	vasopressin
Maintain DO_2 level	Raise in pump flow
272 ml/min/m^2	Raise Hb level
	Raise O_2 sat
	Decrease body temp
Support graft	Milrinone (0.2–0.5 mcg/kg/min)
	Dopamine (4–6 mcg/kg/min)
	Epinephrine (0.05–0.25 mcg/kg/min)
Hb level	11 g/dl
Maintain regular rhythm	K$^+$/Mg$^+$
and A-V synchrony	Pacing
110 bpm	Isoprenaline (0.02–0.04 mcg/kg/min)
Pacing with 110–120 bpm	Increase of HR increases CI, avoid overload
Reduce PVR (if necessary)	iNO (20–40 ppm)
	Inhalatory iloprost (10–20 ng)
	Inhalatory milrinone (5 mg) for 15 min
Slowly reduce CPB flow (careful monitoring CVP, TEE, LAP)	Check/change drug infusion rate
	Check chamber filling
	Check contractility

Table 3. Practice guide to wean from CPB.

Drug	Average dosage	Advantages	Side effects
Epinephrine	0.05–0.25 mcg/kg/min	Support RV overload	Tachycardia, arrhythmias, raise O_2 demand
Norepinephrine	Up to 0.15 mcg/kg/min	Contrast vasodilatation	Increase PVR
Levosimendan	0.1–0.2 mcg/kg/min	Support RV overload	Vasodilation
Milrinone	0.2–0.5 mcg/kg/min	Support RV overload	Arrhythmias, raise O_2 demand, vasodilation
Vasopressin	2.5–5 U/h	Contrast vasodilatation	Increase SVR impair forward flow of LVAD
i-NO	20–40 ppm	Reduce PVR (if not fixed)	
i-Milrinone	5 mg/15 min	Reduce PVR (if not fixed)	
i-Iloprost	20–30 mcg/15 min	Reduce PVR (if not fixed)	
Methylene blue	0.5–2 mg/kg	Contrast vasodilation	

Table 4. Inotropes/vasoactive: average therapeutic dosage to support hemodynamics.

Inotropic score	Dopamine (µg/kg/min) + dobutamine (µg/kg/min) + 100 × epinephrine (µg/kg/min)
Vasoactive inotropic score (modified by Davidson et al. with inclusion of vasoactive medication	IS + 10 × milrinone (µg/kg/min) + 10 × vasopressin (U/kg/min) + 100 × norepinephrine (µg/kg/min
Vasoactive inotropic score plus levosimendan	VIS + 10 × levosimendan (mcg/kg/min)
Poor clinical outcome	VIS 20–24 (in the first 24 h) + VIS 15–19 (in the subsequent 24 h)

Table 5. Inotropic score.

IAS (interatrial septum) or "fluttering" of IVS (interventricular septum) during end-diastole, TAPSE(tricuspid annular plane systolic excursion), and MPI (myocardial performance index).

Basic ventilation strategies to reduce pulmonary artery resistances such as hyperoxia and moderate hyperventilation are mandatory. Ventilation should be set at 60–100% FiO_2, 6–8 ml/kg TV (tidal volume), and low-moderate PEEP (5–6 cmH_2O), after recruitment maneuver, with the intention to prevent lung atelectasis [12].

Chest closure can be very critical for hemodynamics. In some rare cases (i.e., 2.5%), primary graft failure can occur [13], and it is responsible for more than 30% of early deaths after cardiac transplantation. Clinical onset of primary graft failure is with hypotension, low cardiac output, high preload pressures (PVC, LAP, and wedge pressure), and biventricular failure. When necessary, a temporary IABP (intra-aortic balloon pump), as first step, and then peripheral (femoral vein-femoral artery) or central (left atrium, right atrium, aorta) VA-ECMO (venous-arteriosus extracorporeal membrane oxygenation) should be taken into account, whenever hemodynamics remain unsatisfactory despite high inotropic support (**Table 5**) [14].

4. Fluid management

Fluid management should be "goal directed," that is, guided by the above-mentioned hemodynamic and echocardiographic parameters, and with the aim to avoid a fluid overload, which is very harmful for the lungs and the right ventricle, while providing adequate intravascular space filling. This should be done via balanced colloids and crystalloids in order to avoid electrolyte disorders and hyperchloremic hyperkalemic metabolic acidosis. Adequate oxygen delivery is ensured by maintaining the hemoglobin level around 10–11 g/dL and an adequate plasma oncotic power is ensured by giving the right amount of albumin.

5. Anticoagulation and hemostasis

To go on CPB, we need to provide an appropriate anticoagulation via unfractionated heparin (300–400 U/kg). A value of ACT at least of 480 s is enough to start the extracorporeal circulation. In case of low response to a full dose of heparin, we can achieve an adequate ACT by administering antithrombin III (AT3), especially when AT3 plasma levels are less than 70%. From 0.5 to 5% of patients with end-stage heart disease can develop HIT (heparin-induced thrombocytopenia), due to repeated heparin exposures related to the placement of IABP, LVADs, or frequent catheter procedures. Alternative anticoagulation, with direct thrombin inhibitors (bivalirudin and argatroban), [8] is recommended in such patients. At the end of organ implantation, once the aortic and right atrium cannulas are removed, we need to guarantee an appropriate heparin reversal with protamine (50 mg of protamine every 50 mg of heparin). We also give the patient 2 g of tranexamic acid at the induction of general anesthesia and 2 g (25–50 mg/kg) with protamine in association with 1 g of gluconate calcium, to avoid hyperfibrinolysis and replace calcium deficiency. Severe bleeding is not a rare condition especially in patients with previous heart surgery. Particularly, in patients with LVADs as bridge to transplant, severe bleeding can often occur due to the large wound area and pretreatment with multiple anticoagulants and platelet inhibitors. If hemostasis is insufficient and the patient is still bleeding, we need to check for coagulation disorders via ROTEM (i.e., hyperfibrinolysis, coagulation factor deficiency, and hypofibrinogenemia) or via TEG and correct the specific deficiency (prothrombin complex concentrate for clotting factor deficiency or fibrinogen concentrate for hypofibrinogenemia). We prefer this approach instead of large dose of fresh frozen plasma, in order to avoid TACO (transfusion-associated circulatory overload), TRALI (transfusion-related lung injury), immune modulation, and increased risk of infections.

6. Intensive care management

Almost 90% of heart transplants are due to ischemic or dilatative cardiomyopathy and men over 40 years of age are the most involved. They all need a special care and a multimodal approach, even because not only cardiovascular balance but also respiratory care, fluid management, and immune system modulation impact on the overall survival.

6.1. ICU admission

Patients incoming from the operating room have to be placed in an isolated single bed room to avoid contamination, since they will undergo immunosuppressive therapy. Everyone in contact with them must wear mask, cup, and sterile gown and do routine sterile hand washing. Invasive hemodynamic monitoring, including systemic arterial pressure, right atrial pressure, pulmonary artery pressure through the PAC, and left atrial pressure, should be immediately reconnected in the room.

Twelve lead ECG at the arrival is mandatory to check heart rhythm disorders. Bradyarrhythmias and supraventricular arrhythmias are the most frequent and should be related to inotropic and chronotropic support, hypovolemia, and electrolyte disorders. If atrial fibrillation occurs, an acute rejection should be considered and a 500 mg bolus of methylprednisolone should be administered, eventually followed by amiodarone (300 mg iv bolus in 30 min) for pharmacological cardioversion and rate control. In case of failure of pharmacological cardioversion, we can try electrical cardioversion. Sinus bradycardia can be treated with low-dose isoprenaline (0.01–0.04 mcg/kg/min), adrenaline (0.01–0.04 mcg/kg/min), and/or temporary atrial pacing, in order to ensure a heart rate about 100–110 bpm. In case of severe AV block, a sequential pacing is required. Anyway, if the patient is still pacing dependent after 2 weeks from the operation, implantation of a permanent pace maker should be considered. Then, you can proceed to request chest X-ray to check the lungs, endotracheal and nasogastric tube position, chest drains, and intravascular devices (CVP line, PAC, and pacing wires) and send for laboratory tests including standard coagulation, renal and liver function, platelets, red blood cell and white blood cell counts, troponin I, CK, albumin, viral markers, thyroid markers, and glycaemia. Blood samples should be sent for good practice also for coagulation tests (ROTEM or TEG) in case of excessive bleeding. A plan for immunosuppressive therapy (methylprednisolone, thymoglobulins, etc.) must be provided in collaboration with specialist immunologist and cardiologist. Antibiotic therapy must be tailored on the background history of donor and/or recipient.

7. Hemodynamic management

Hemodynamic stability, after heart transplant, may be impaired by several pathophysiological processes, including autonomic denervation, with subsequent chronotropic and inotropic failure, ischemia reperfusion injury, metabolic acidosis, and volume depletion. To support such effects, several endpoints must be taken into account:

7.1. Intravascular volume optimization

A goal-directed therapy is the ideal way to ensure adequate fluid filling. It means using the above-mentioned hemodynamic parameters coming from invasive monitoring and from echocardiographic evaluation, to be guided in the fluid replacement. Once the need of fluids is clear, the physician should decide the most ideal fluid in order to avoid peripheral organ oncotic damage (i.e., hyperoncotic kidney failure from hydroxyethyl starches [15]); hyperchloremic hyperkalemic acidosis, which can impact itself on kidney function; and fluid overload into the interstitial space. Crystalloids have a less oncotic power than colloids; however, albumin can cross the pulmonary capillary membrane, if damaged, and anyway it can recirculate through the pulmonary barrier 24 hours from the administration: then balanced crystalloids and balanced colloids (albumin solution at 5 or 20%) should be given at the right per kilo amount and the fluid responsiveness should be tested while they are given.

7.2. Narrow monitoring of hemodynamic parameters

During the recovery period (approximately 7–14 days), a narrow monitoring of hemodynamic and vital parameters is mandatory: IBP, CI, CO, ISVRI, IPVR, PAPs, HR, SvO_2, LAP/PCWP, TPG, SpO_2, ECG, body temperature, urine output, and lactate levels.

Target values are: CVP ≤ 12 mmHg, MAP > 65 mmHg, LAP 8–12 mmHg, SvO_2 over 65%, HR about 100–110 bpm, urine output > 1.5 ml/kg, and lactate < 2 mmol/L.

7.3. Pharmacological support

The goal is to ensure adequate CO, avoiding excessive increase of cardiac preload and afterload, while maintaining adequate heart rate. Chronotropic support is achieved through low-moderate dose of isoprenaline or by atrial-sequential external pacing. Inotropic effect is achieved through moderate-high dose of adrenaline and, when necessary, with phosphodiesterase inhibitors as milrinone that also decreases peripheral vascular resistances. Other pharmacological tools that are aimed to control arterial ventricle coupling are nitroglycerin and sodium nitroprusside, very helpful to decrease the afterload of the left ventricle and increase cardiac output, when used together with an inotropic drug. In case of preexistent pulmonary hypertension, inhalation of nitric oxide and imbrication with sildenafil can help to reduce pulmonary vascular resistances [14]. In the further postoperative course, addition of an upstream therapy including ace inhibitors, b-blockers, or calcium antagonists may be helpful as cardiac protection.

7.4. Support the right ventricle of the donor heart

The donor heart, particularly the right ventricle, in case of preexisting precapillary or postcapillary pulmonary hypertension, has to fight with high afterload [**Table 6**]. The preexisting conditions may be impaired in case of coexisting hypoxia or hypercapnia, prolonged extracorporeal circulation, and donor ischemia with consequent ischemia-reperfusion injury, blood transfusion, and protamine administration. Right ventricular failure may be challenging and really impacts on the overall survival of transplanted patients [18].

Early PA pressure monitoring at the time of CPB weaning is fundamental and has to be continued in the early postoperative period. The first aim in hemodynamic management of the graft is to offload the right ventricle, decreasing PA pressures and pulmonary vascular resistances while ensuring an adequate RV contractility. Inhaled nitric oxide at 20–40 ppm is a rapid onset tool to decrease PA pressures. It seems to improve early clinical outcomes in heart transplanted patients, but literature is still lacking in terms of overall survival [9].

This is the reason why it is often used preventively during weaning from the CPB. Alternatively, the prostacyclin analog iloprost (6 × 5–10 mcg) can be given.

After the very early postoperative period, inhaled nitric oxide can be substituted by the phosphodiesterase-5 inhibitor sildenafil at the dosage of 20 mg × 3/die via NG tube with very small effects on the systemic pressures, avoiding also the rebound phenomena coming from the discontinuation of inhaled nitric oxide therapy. Sildenafil has also been shown to decrease PA pressures during inhalation of nitric oxide, since they seem to activate different regulatory mechanisms of the vascular tone [19, 20]. Inotropic support of the RV should be guaranteed by moderate-high dose of adrenaline (0.05–0.1 mcg/kg/min) or low-moderate doses of phosphodiesterase inhibitors as milrinone (0.2–0.3 mcg/kg/min).

Clearly, while supporting the right ventricle, we need to ensure adequate oxygenation, avoid hypercapnia, maintain adequate lung recruitment by PEEP (not over 6 cmH$_2$O), and guarantee a negative fluid balance in order to reduce the preload and optimize the afterload [**Table 6**]. If all these maneuvers are not sufficient, we have to consider a temporary mechanical right ventricle support via peripheral VA-ECMO.

Monitor by PAC	CVP, MPAP, PCWP, CO, SvO$_2$
Mechanical ventilation	PaO$_2$ 100 mmHg, pCO$_2$ 30–35 mmHg, pH 7.5. Adequate peep level (5–10 cm H$_2$O) to recruit lung and optimize PVR
Restricted fluid therapy	Monitoring filling pressure CVP 10–12 mmHg, PCWP 12–15 mmHg
	Monitoring LVEDV, RVEDV by echocardiography
Inotropes to support RV contractility	Epinephrine 0.02–0.25 mcg/kg/min
Inodilator	Milrinone 0.2–0.5 mcg/kg/min
	Levosimendan 0.2 mcg/kg/min ± norepinephrine (up to 0.15 mcg/kg/min) to maintain right coronary perfusion pressure
iNO	5–40 ppm
Phosphodiesterase V inhibitor	Revatio 3 × 20 mg p.o.
Systemic vasodilators	Sodium nitroprusside, prostacyclin PGI$_2$ analogon iloprost (2 ng/kg/min)

Table 6. Pulmonary artery hypertension monitoring and right ventricular dysfunction prevention.

In case of concomitant LV insufficiency and signs of systemic hypoperfusion (with raising of LAP/PCWP and sudden reduction of CO, CI, and SvO$_2$), we will need to increase the inotrope support and try to compensate the peripheral vasoconstriction with peripheral vasodilators as nitroprusside, when the MAPs allow to do that, in order to reduce left ventricle afterload and facilitate the ejection. The conditioning with inodilators as levosimendan [10] can be very helpful and, in case of massive peripheral vasodilatory response, it can be compensated with mean dosage of noradrenaline to ensure adequate MAPs. When this is not enough, an additional support with IABP should be considered, but, when insufficient, a central or peripheral VA-ECMO will be placed. The simultaneous presence of the IABP will help avoid pulmonary edema by reducing the afterload of LV.

7.5. Avoid metabolic acidosis and monitor acid-base balance and kidney function

A patient undergoing heart transplant comes from a long period of low cardiac output, so the kidney dysfunction is often preexisting.

In the immediate postoperative period, urinary output may decrease for several reasons including intravascular volume depletion and kidney damage coming from long lasting extracorporeal support or from the use of unbalanced solutions for fluid challenge. In addition, a high use of colloidal molecules may damage directly the renal tubules with a process called "osmotic-nephrosis." If urine output is <0.5 ml/kg/h despite optimization of blood pressure, preload and CO, and use of standard diuretics (furosemide or torasemide), and the patient develops kidney failure with serum urea >200 mg/dL or hyperkalemia, kidney replacement therapy becomes mandatory.

We prefer early application of continuous venovenous hemofiltration (CVVH) for a complete hemodynamic and fluid rebalancing. In case kidney replacement therapy is necessary in a long-term postoperative period, the change is made to intermittent dialysis (three times weekly).

7.6. Consider echocardiography as a main tool, together with PAC, to guide hemodynamic management, inotropic support, and fluid challenge

At first, we may exclude significant pericardial collection, assess left ventricle diastolic function of the new performing heart, related to its stiffness and hypertrophy, and think about which wedge pressure we are expected to find [21]. If the systolic function of the new heart is failing, we should exclude an acute graft rejection. Regarding the right ventricle, we must know the recipient preoperative pulmonary vascular resistances, if pre- or postcapillary pulmonary hypertension persists and if it is reversible with phosphodiesterase inhibitors.

RV dysfunction is identified early with a dilation of the right chambers, alteration of interventricular septum movement, and appearance of tricuspid valve insufficiency.

8. Respiratory weaning

A patient undergoing heart transplant should remain under mechanical ventilation until hemodynamic stability is ensured, lactate levels are stable, and immunosuppressive therapy is started. To protect the lungs, we have to limit peak pressures and use low tidal volumes (6 ml/kg) with adequate PEEP level (at least 3–5 cmH$_2$O).

However, disadvantages coming from permissive hypercapnia on the pulmonary vascular resistances and right ventricle afterload, myocardial function, and renal blood flow loads must be taken into account [16]. As a consequence, there are no universal evidences, but the choice must be tailored for the patient. The only certainty is we must avoid hypercapnia, hypoxia, and PEEP over 10 cmH$_2$O and keep peak pressure under 35–40 cmH$_2$O.

During mechanical ventilation, inhaled nitric oxide can be administered in order to reduce right PA pressures, pulmonary vascular resistances, and then right ventricle afterload, especially in the first 24 hours from CPB weaning at the maximum dosage of 20–40 ppm [17, 18]. Once mechanical ventilation is discontinued, inhaled nitric oxide can be substituted by iv or oral pulmonary vasodilators as sildenafil. The weaning criteria do not differ from those used in normal cardiosurgical patients, and the goal is the same: maintain adequate analgesia and sedation levels and wean the patient from the mechanical ventilation as soon as possible. If this is not possible, due to unstable hemodynamics, high inotropic score, respiratory failure, or neurological issues, a percutaneous dilatation tracheostomy will be packaged without further delay (within the first 5–7 days of mechanical ventilation).

Once the patient is awake and self-breathing and the LAP line is removed (generally 24–48 hours from surgery), the patient will need physiotherapy and mobilization.

Early feeding is important. It is initially given via NG tube (25–30 kcal/kg/day) and then self-feeding is achieved once there is no more gastrointestinal paresis.

9. Infection control

Standard prophylaxis is due to cefuroxime 2 g iv every 6 hours in the first 24 hours from heart transplantation (the first two boluses are given in the operating room, at the induction of general anesthesia and once CPB is started). The amount of antibiotic given in the ICU should be tailored for the patient's creatinine clearance, especially if the patient is not under renal filter. Further extension and change of antibiotic therapy should depend on microbiological results of the donor and on microbiological samples of the recipient once admitted in the ICU. Furthermore, in case of redo-operation with existing wound infection, the patient will receive vancomycin and meropenem as standard medication and vancomycin plasma levels should be tested daily. Obviously, due to the immunosuppressive therapy, transplanted patients are very prone to infections. Delivery of care should be done in sterile conditions and, besides standard iv antibiotic therapy, topical antifungal medications should be given in the early postoperative period.

10. Immunosuppressive therapy

A specific team is taking care of immunosuppressive therapy. It starts with 500 mg iv bolus of solumedrol at the CPB weaning. Once admitted in the ICU, the patient will receive 125 mg bolus of solumedrol every 8 hours, with a specific descending dose scheme.

Antithymocyte globulines (1.5 mg/kg iv) are usually given 4, 24, and 48 hours after the end of the transplantation. They will be adjusted based on eventual presence of high body temperature, bleeding, and thrombocytopenia. There are several possible immunosuppressive agents that will be tailored for the patient such as tacrolimus, cyclosporin A, everolimus, and mycophenolate.

11. Graft dysfunction

An international consensus conference in 2014 has classified the graft dysfunction into primary graft dysfunction (PDG) and secondary graft dysfunction (SGD). The first one occurs 24 h from heart transplant and can involve the left, the right ventricle, or both, with different degrees of dysfunction. Typical signs are severe deficit of systolic function, low cardiac output, and high filling pressures without evidence of acute graft rejection or cardiac tamponade. The SGD has a specific reason such as acute rejection, pulmonary hypertension, or surgical complications. Risk factors to develop PGD may be related to the recipient, donor, or technical factors [22].

Donor-related risk factors may be:

- Age (increased risk of 20% every decade)
- Sex (nearly doubled risk with female)

Recipient-related risk factors may be:

- High vasoactive or inotropic support (doubled risk)
- Uncontrolled diabetes (doubled risk)

Technical risk factors are:

- Warm ischemic time (= explant time + implant time); implant time was found to be a strong predictor of PGD.
- Resternotomy (it has been identified as a risk factor for severe PGD due to adherences and tissue fibrosis that can extend the explant time and increase the risk of infections).
- Prolonged CPB time, with subsequent systemic inflammatory response, vasoplegia, clotting and platelet dysfunction, leukocyte activation, free oxygen radical release, and larger amount of blood products given.

All these factors can increase the ischemic-reperfusion injury and the overall mortality [23].

The first step to treat a PDG is vasoactive and inotropic support. If it were not sufficient, an intra-aortic balloon pump (IABP) placement may help.

In case of very severe PGD, an extracorporeal membrane oxygenation (ECMO) becomes the only emergency treatment.

11.1. Anesthesia and intensive care management

11.1.1. For cardiac transplantation in pediatrics

Pediatric heart transplant represents a small subgroup (14%) of total cardiac transplant where the differences in anatomy and physiology make the surgical procedure and the management more complex and creates a unique scenario [24].

The management of pediatric patients undergoing cardiac transplantation differs from the adult patients because it requires a specific knowledge of physiology and physiopathology at different stages of growth, from the newborns through childhood up to adulthood.

This heterogeneous population with a wide range of age, genetic disorders, anatomical anomalies, and symptoms can be classified in four different groups based on the different etiology: 1—CHD (congenital heart disease); 2—DCM (dilated cardiomyopathy); 3—RETX (retransplant); 4—OTHER (**Table 7**) [25]; each of these has specific features.

11.1.2. Preoperative evaluation

The preoperative evaluation is an essential step in order to better analyze both the cardiac pathology and the possible related comorbidities.

Category (abbreviation)	Diagnoses in category
Congenital heart disease (CHD)	Congenital heart defects: HLHS-unoperated, with surgery, without surgery, valvular heart disease
Dilated cardiomyopathy (DCM)	Dilated myopathy due to alcohol, familiar, idiopathic, myocarditis, viral, postpartum, etc.
Retransplant (RETX)	Due to acute rejection, coronary artery disease, etc.
Other (OTHER)	Arrhythmogenic right ventricular dysplasia, cancer, coronary artery disease, myopathy-ischemia, hypertrophic cardiomyopathy, etc.

Table 7. Diagnosis for pediatric heart transplant.

Main preoperative features and examinations that must be considered are:

- Type of heart disease (CHD, DCM, RETX, and OTHER)

- Right heart catheterization (RHC): pulmonary artery pressure (PAP), pulmonary capillary wedge pressure (PCWP), pulmonary vascular resistances (PVR), and pulmonary hypertension etiology. Unfortunately, most patients with congenital heart defects have high PVR because of pulmonary vascular disease. However, the presence of systemic-to-pulmonary shunts, intra-pulmonary shunting, and caval pulmonary circulation does not allow a correct assessment of PVR. For these patients, RHC should be performed at 3–6 month interval in adult patients but is not advocated as routine surveillance in children unless a clinical change is noted [26].

- Numbers and types of previous operations (sternotomy and thoracotomy).

- Cyanotic congenital heart disease (secondary erythrocytosis, hyperviscosity, and coagulation deficit).

- Panel reactive antibody (PRA) identifies sensitized patients. It may be elevated in patients with allograft patch or with multiple redo-operations, due to the multiple transfusions. It may result in an increased risk of acute rejection [27].

- Variable anatomic substrates (isomerism, issues of situs, MAPCAs, aberrant right or left subclavian artery, and persistence of left superior vena cava).

- Previous venous or arterial thromboembolism (central venous catheter thrombosis).

- Previous neurological history: syncope, previous stroke, and cerebral arteriovenous malformation.

- Respiratory insufficiency: smoke, chronic obstructive pulmonary disease (COPD), anatomical anomalies of the pulmonary vessels, and presence of bronchial or pulmonary stents.

- Arrhythmias and previous ICD implantation.

- Liver disease: an evaluation of the patient's liver profile is extremely important. Chronic heart failure and in particular the univentricular heart physiology can lead to a liver dysfunction.

Fontan-associated liver disease (FALD) is a liver dysfunction due to a chronic elevated central venous pressure, low cardiac output, persistent hypoxemia, and intrahepatic venous thrombosis. FALD can be expressed in different stages, from moderate hepatic congestion up to liver cirrhosis with portal hypertension. In several cases, liver function is preserved or is only slightly altered, with high international normalizer ratio (INR), low factor V levels, and elevated factor VIII levels [28].

- Kidney disease: acute or acute-on-chronic renal dysfunction.

- Coagulation anomalies may be present as result of chronic anticoagulation, liver disease, or as a result of cyanotic congenital heart disease (reduced levels of coagulation factors II, V, VII, IX, and X, accelerated fibrinolysis, and fibrinogen alterations).

- Gastrointestinal disorders: necrotizing enterocolitis in newborns or protein losing enteropathy (PLE), which is an excessive protein loss through the gastrointestinal tract that can be present after Fontan operation (even if its origins are poorly understood) [29]

12. Intraoperative management

The anesthetic management should consider that these patients have a poor cardiac reserve and that the premedication, general anesthesia, and the surgical manipulation after the sternotomy can lead to a destabilization of the hemodynamics.

Antibiotic therapy differs according to age and weight and background of both the donor and recipient (**Tables 8** and **9**).

Immunosuppression is started 1 hour before going to the operating room: thymoglobulin 1 mg/kg/12 h and methylprednisolone 7–10 mg/kg (max. 125 mg).

Premedication is performed, according to clinical condition, with low doses of benzodiazepines (midazolam 0.3–0.5 mg/kg orally or rectal in neonate) avoiding excessive sedation and consequently hypercapnia.

It is well known that in newborns and infants, placing an invasive monitoring before induction of anesthesia is not always possible; therefore, it is essential to have a noninvasive monitoring before starting the drug administration.

General anesthesia is induced by inhalation of sevoflurane/desflurane in newborns and infants and by intravenous injections of midazolam 0.3–0.5 mg/kg, fentanyl 2–4 mcg/kg, rocuronium 1 mg/kg, and propofol 2–4 mg/kg in adults and children. Moreover, for continuous infusion of the anesthesia, propofol 4–6 mg/kg/h in adults, while midazolam 0.2 mg/kg/h and fentanyl 2 mcg/kg/h in newborns and children are recommended. After induction, hydrocortisone 10–20 mg/kg is infused.

In all patients, regional cerebral monitoring is achieved with the use of near infrared spectroscopy (NIRS).

Newborn < 1200 g	20 mg q 12 h
Newborn ≥ 1200 g < 7 days of life	20 mg q 12 h
Newborn ≥ 1200 gr > 7 days of life	20 mg q 8 h
Infants and children	100 mg/kg/24 h in 3 doses

Table 8. Antibiotic therapy (cefazolin).

Newborn < 1200 g	5 mg q 12 h
Newborn = 2000 g < 7 days of life	5 mg q 12 h
Newborn = 2000 g > 7 days of life	5 mg q 8 h
Newborn > 2000 g < 7 days of life	5 mg q 8 h
Newborn > 2000 g > 7 days of life	5 mg q 6 h
Infants and children	15/40 mg/kg/24 h in 3–4 doses

In case of allergy to beta-lactams, clindamycin is administered.

Table 9. Antibiotic therapy (clindamycin).

Different conditions may complicate the venous central catheter placing as: anatomical variables, possible occlusion due to previous repeated catheterizations, and previous positioning of central lines. In these cases, the echo-guided assistance is recommended. In smaller patients or in occluded jugular/subclavian veins, femoral veins can be also used. The sizing of the catheter and the numbers of lumens used depend on the weight and age of the patients. When possible, a pulmonary artery catheter (PAC) must be placed into the superior vena cava and then correctly repositioned by the cardiac surgeon before removing the aortic cross-clamp. In newborns and infants, placing PAC may be problematic or impossible due to the size of the patient. In these cases, it is possible to use the central venous oxygen saturation (SCvO$_2$) as a surrogate of SVO$_2$ even if the results are controversial [30].

As an alternative, the left atrial pressure (LAP) can be monitored with the insertion of a catheter through the right superior pulmonary vein.

Transesophageal echocardiography (TEE) is always recommended for a correct evaluation of biventricular function, after the CPB weaning, accordingly with the patient's weight.

After induction of the anesthesia, the ventilation management requires extreme attention since the hypoxia and the hypercapnia can increase PVR leading to a low cardiac output syndrome. In case of hypotension, before infusing, a bolus of colloid is essential to secure the correct ventilation, avoiding respiratory acidosis.

The majority of patients with CHD undergoing cardiac transplantation are reoperation candidates, so it is important to put into account long operative times, due to dissection of the adhesions and complex reconstruction of the anatomy.

12.1. CPB and weaning

CPB management can be extremely complex and differs according to the patient's weight and age. The main aim is to maintain a correct medium arterial pressure (MAP) and a correct DO_2/VO_2 ratio.

Sometimes, this is difficult to be achieved, due to the possible presence of anatomical extra-cardiac shunts. The dose of unfractionated heparin for the CPB is 200 U/kg in newborns and infants or 300 U/kg in the child and adult, in order to have an ACT > 400 s. In case of reduced response to heparin, administration of ATIII at a dose of 100 mg/kg is recommended. Furthermore, in case of HIT or low response to heparin, direct thrombin inhibitors are administered (bivalirudin and argatroban) as in adult patients. After the aortic cross-clamp is removed, methylprednisolone is administered with the dose of 7–10 mg/kg (max. 125 mg/kg).

Weaning from CPB always requires inotropic support and the right ventricular failure is a possible complication, characterized by restrictive pattern that can be managed by inhaled nitric oxide (5–40 ppm) and inotropic support (milrinone 0.3–0.75 mcg/kg/min, adrenaline 0.02–0.1 mcg/kg/min, and isoprenaline 0.1–1 mcg/kg/min) in order to vasodilate the pulmonary circulation improving biventricular contractility and providing a chronotropic effect if bradycardia occurs. It is extremely important to keep normal PVR by providing a proper ventilation, avoiding hypoxia and maintaining normocapnia.

Once the patient has been weaned form CBP, the vigilance or $SCvO_2$ can monitor the hemodynamic profile and biventricular function can be evaluated with echocardiogram.

However, in case of poor CO, despite maximal inotropic support and correct ventilation, we should consider the support via an extracorporeal membrane oxygenation (ECMO).

12.2. Anticoagulation and hemostasis

At the end of CPB, heparin is antagonized with a ratio 2:1 or 1:1 with protamine based on the ACT values. Antifibrinolytic agents are administrated at the dosage of 50 mg/kg (25 mg/kg after general anesthesia induction and 25 mg/kg at the end of CPB). Severe bleeding is not uncommon in pediatric population. Main reasons of postoperative bleeding are previous heart surgery, cyanotic congenital heart disease, immature coagulation system, and excessive hemodilution due to the disproportionate ratio of CPB circuit volume to patient blood volume, especially in newborns and infants. Correct coagulation management is always achieved through ROTEM.

12.3. Intensive care

During the postoperative intensive care course, close monitoring of hemodynamic parameters, inotropes, ventilation, and acid base balance is required to predict pulmonary hypertension, biventricular failure, and LCOS. Normalization of the oxygenation and ventilation is the primary goal in these patients and ventilation support must be discontinued as soon as possible. The antibiotic therapy will be set according to microbiological surveillance. Immunotherapy during the postoperative course is managed by the cardiologist as follows: methylprednisolone, thymoglobulin, tacrolimus, and mycophenolate.

12.4. Peculiar problems

In the postoperative setting, the main problems for pediatric patients are comorbidities related to chronic decompensation and univentricular physiology.

- Cyanotic congenital heart disease: patients with long standing hypoxemia often develop severe alteration of whole blood viscosity and alteration of coagulation profiles with high risk of postoperative bleeding [31].

- Plastic bronchitis: it is a rare complication of univentricular physiology characterized by the formation of exudative airway casts that can occlude airways and cause respiratory failure. The etiology is still not well identified, but it seems to relate to an increased central venous pressure or lymphatic drainage alterations [32].

- Protein losing enteropathy (PLE): it is defined as a possible complication of the univentricular circulation. It can arise after the Fontan operation (5–15% of the patients) [33]. It is characterized by the abnormal loss of proteins into the enteral lumen, which results in hypoproteinemia and hypoalbuminemia. This leads to an increase of lymphatic drainage and a dilation of intestinal lymphatic system with an impaired fat absorption resulting in steatorrhea. Moreover, the hypoproteinemia may result also in ascites, peripheral edema, and pleural/pericardial effusion. Therapy consists of diuretics, corticosteroids, and albumin supplementation.

Abbreviations

BIS	bispectral index
CI	cardiac index
CO	cardiac output
COPD	chronic obstructive pulmonary disease
CPB	cardiopulmonary bypass
CVC	central venous catheter
CVP	central venous pressure
CVVH	central venovenous hemofiltration
DLCO	carbon monoxide lung diffusion
ECMO	extracorporeal membranous oxygenation
HIT	heparin-induced thrombocytopenia
IABP	intra-aortic balloon pump
ICD	implantable cardioverter defibrillator

ISVR	indexed systemic vascular resistance
LAP	left atrial pressure
LV	left ventricle
LVAD	left ventricular assist device
NGT	nasogastric tube
NO	nitrogen oxide
OCS	organ care system
PAC	pulmonary artery catheter
PAP	pulmonary arterial pressure
PCWP	pulmonary capillary wedge pressure
PEEP	positive end expiratory pressure
PPM	parts per millions
PGD	primary graft dysfunction
PVR	pulmonary vascular resistance
RAP	right atrial pressure
RV	right ventricle
SIRS	systemic inflammatory response syndrome
SVR	systemic vascular resistance
TACO	transfusion-associated circulatory overload
TPG	transpulmonary pressure gradient
TRALI	transfusion-associated lung injury
TV	tidal volume
VAD	ventricular assist device
WU	wood unit

Author details

Massimo Baiocchi*, Maria Benedetto, Marta Agulli and Guido Frascaroli

*Address all correspondence to: massimo.baiocchi@aosp.bo.it

Anaesthesiology and Intensive Care Unit, Cardiothoracic and vascular Department, Policlinico S. Orsola University Hospital, Bologna, Italy

References

[1] Mehra MR, Kobashigawa J, Starling R, et al. Listing criteria for heart transplantation: International Society for Heart and Lung Transplantation guidelines for the care of cardiac transplant candidates – 2006. The Journal of Heart and Lung Transplantation. 2006;**25**:1024-1042

[2] Miller WL, Grill DE, Borlaug BA. Clinical features, hemodynamics, and outcomes of pulmonary hypertension due to chronic heart failure with reduced ejection fraction: Pulmonary hypertension and heart failure. JACC: Heart Failure. 2013;**1**:290-299

[3] Lundgren J, Soderlund C, et al. Impact of postoperative pulmonary hypertension on outcome after heart transplantation. Scandinavian Cardiovascular Journal. 2017; **51**(3):172-181

[4] de Groote P, El Sri C, Fertin M. Sildenafil in heart transplant candidates with pulmonary hypertension. Archives of Cardiovascular Diseases. 2015;**108**(6-7):375-384. DOI: 10.1016/j.acvd.2015.01.013

[5] Micha Z, Pacholewicz J, Copik I. Mechanical circulatory support is effective to treat pulmonary hypertension in heart transplant candidates disqualified due to unacceptable pulmonary vascular resistance. Kardiochir Torakochirurgia Pol. 2018;**15**(1):23-26

[6] Waterman PM, Bjerke R. Rapid-sequence induction technique in patients with severe ventricular dysfunction. Journal of Cardiothoracic Anesthesia. 1988;**2**:602-606

[7] Stobierska-Dzierzek B, Awead H, Michler RE. The evolving management of acute right-sided heart failure in cardiac transplant recipients. Journal of the American College of Cardiology. 2001;**38**:923-931

[8] Levy JH, Winkler AM. Heparin-induced thrombocytopenia and cardiac surgery. Current Opinion in Anaesthesiology. 2010;**23**:74-79

[9] Benedetto M, Romano R, et al. Inhaled nitric oxide in cardiac surgery: Evidence or tradition? Nitrix Oxide. 2015;**49**:67-69

[10] Weis F, Beiras-Fernandez A, Kaczmarek I, et al. Levosimendan: A new therapeutic option in the treatment of primary graft dysfunction after heart transplantation. The Journal of Heart and Lung Transplantation. 2009;**28**:501-504

[11] Landoni G, Lomivorotov VV, Alvaro G, et al. Levosimendan for hemodynamic support after cardiac surgery. The New England Journal of Medicine. 2017;**25**:2021-2031

[12] Koster A, Diehl C, Dongas A, et al. Anesthesia for cardiac transplantation: A practical overview of current management strategies. Applied Cardiopulmonary Pathophysiology. 2011;**15**:213-219

[13] Kirk R, Edwards LB, Kucheryavaya AY, et al. The registry of the International Society for Heart and Lung Transplantation: Fourteenth pediatric heart transplantation report-2011. The Journal of Heart and Lung Transplantation. 2011;**30**:1095-1103

[14] Costanzo MR, Taylor D, Hunt S, et al. The International Society of Heart and Lung Transplantation guideline for the care of heart transplant recipients. The Journal of Heart and Lung Transplantation. 2010;**29**:914-956

[15] Rioux JP, Lessard M, De Bortolli B, Roy P, Albert M, Verdant C, et al. Pentastarch 10% (250 kDa/0.45) is and independent risk factor of acute kidney injury following cardiac surgery. Critical Care Medicine. 2009;**37**(4):1293-1298

[16] The Acute Respiratory Distress Syndrome Network. Ventilation with lower tidal volumes as compared with traditional tidal volumes for acute lung injury and the acute respiratory distress syndrome. The New England Journal of Medicine. 2000;**342**:1301-1308

[17] Ardehali A, Hughes K, Sadeghi A, Esmailian D, Marelli D, et al. Inhaled nitric oxide for pulmonary hypertension after heart transplantation. Transplantation. 2001;**72**:638-641

[18] Kaul TK, Fields BL. Postoperative acute refractory right ventricular failure: Incidence, pathogenesis, management and prognosis. Cardivascular Surgery. 2000;**8**:1-9

[19] Atz AM, Lefler AK, Fairbrother DL, Uber WE, et al. Sildefanil augments the effect of inhaled nitric oxide for postoperative pulmonary hypertensive crises. The Journal of Thoracic and Cardiovascular Surgery. 2002;**124**:628-629

[20] Ghofrani HA, Wiedemann R, Rose F, Schermuly RT, et al. Combination therapy with oral sildenafil and inhaled iloprost for severe pulmonary hypertension. Annals of Internal Medicine. 2002;**136**:515-522

[21] Erb JM. Role of echocardiography in intensive care treatment of patients after heart transplantation or implantation of a ventricular assist device. Intensivmedizin und Notfallmedizin. 2006;**43**(5):431-443

[22] Kobashigawa J, Zuckermann A, et al. Report from a consensus conference on primary graft dysfunction after cardiac transplantation. The Journal of Heart and Lung Transplantation. 2014;**33**(4):327.40

[23] Avtaar Singh SS, Banner NR, et al. ISHLT primary graft dysfunction incidence, risk factors and outcome: A UK National Study. Transplantation. 2018;**5**

[24] Pediatric heart transplantation. Journal of Thoracic Disease. 2015;**7**(3):552-559

[25] The Registry of the International Society for Heart and Lung Transplantation. Nineteenth pediatric lung and heart-lung transplantation report—2016; Focus theme: Primary diagnostic indications for transplant. The Journal of Heart and Lung Transplantation. 2016;**35**(10):1196-1205

[26] The 2016 international society for heart lung transplantation listing criteria for heart transplantation: A 10-year update. Journal of Heart and Lung Transplantation. Jan 2016;**35**(1): 1-23. DOI: 10.1016/j.healun.2015.10.023

[27] Heart transplantation in children for end-stage congenital heart disease. Seminars in Thoracic and Cardiovascular Surgery. Pediatric Cardiac Surgery Annual. 2014;**17**:69-76

[28] Fontan-associated liver disease: Implications for heart transplantation. Journal of Heart and Lung Transplantation. 2016;**35**(1):26-33

[29] StrategFontan-associated protein-losing enteropathy and heart transplant: A pediatric heart transplant study analysis. Journal of Heart and Lung Transplantation. 2015; **34**(9):1169-1176

[30] Fiberoptic monitoring of central venous oxygen saturation (Pediasat) in small children undergoing cardiac surgery: Continuous is not continuous. Version3. F1000Research. 2014 Jan 23 [revised 2014 Jun 13];**3**:23. DOI: 10.12688/f1000research.3-23.v3. eCollection 2014

[31] Cyanotic congenital heart disease (CCHD): Focus on hypoxiemia, secondary erythrocytosis, and coagulation alterations. Pediatric Anaesthesia. 2015;**25**:981-989

[32] Plastic bronchitis in patient with Fontan physiology: Review of the literature and preliminary experience with Fontan conversion and cardiac transplantation. World Journal for Pediatric and Congenital Heart Surgery. 2012;**3**(3):364-372

[33] Strategies to treat protein-losing enteropathy. Pediatric Cardiac Surgery Annual of the Seminars in Thoracic and Cardiovascular Surgery. 2002;**5**:3-11

Permissions

All chapters in this book were first published in HT, by InTech Open; hereby published with permission under the Creative Commons Attribution License or equivalent. Every chapter published in this book has been scrutinized by our experts. Their significance has been extensively debated. The topics covered herein carry significant findings which will fuel the growth of the discipline. They may even be implemented as practical applications or may be referred to as a beginning point for another development.

The contributors of this book come from diverse backgrounds, making this book a truly international effort. This book will bring forth new frontiers with its revolutionizing research information and detailed analysis of the nascent developments around the world.

We would like to thank all the contributing authors for lending their expertise to make the book truly unique. They have played a crucial role in the development of this book. Without their invaluable contributions this book wouldn't have been possible. They have made vital efforts to compile up to date information on the varied aspects of this subject to make this book a valuable addition to the collection of many professionals and students.

This book was conceptualized with the vision of imparting up-to-date information and advanced data in this field. To ensure the same, a matchless editorial board was set up. Every individual on the board went through rigorous rounds of assessment to prove their worth. After which they invested a large part of their time researching and compiling the most relevant data for our readers.

The editorial board has been involved in producing this book since its inception. They have spent rigorous hours researching and exploring the diverse topics which have resulted in the successful publishing of this book. They have passed on their knowledge of decades through this book. To expedite this challenging task, the publisher supported the team at every step. A small team of assistant editors was also appointed to further simplify the editing procedure and attain best results for the readers.

Apart from the editorial board, the designing team has also invested a significant amount of their time in understanding the subject and creating the most relevant covers. They scrutinized every image to scout for the most suitable representation of the subject and create an appropriate cover for the book.

The publishing team has been an ardent support to the editorial, designing and production team. Their endless efforts to recruit the best for this project, has resulted in the accomplishment of this book. They are a veteran in the field of academics and their pool of knowledge is as vast as their experience in printing. Their expertise and guidance has proved useful at every step. Their uncompromising quality standards have made this book an exceptional effort. Their encouragement from time to time has been an inspiration for everyone.

The publisher and the editorial board hope that this book will prove to be a valuable piece of knowledge for researchers, students, practitioners and scholars across the globe.

List of Contributors

Hannah Copeland
University of Mississippi Medical Center, Jackson, Mississippi, United States of America

Jack G. Copeland
University of Arizona, Tucson, Arizona, United States of America

Martin Schweiger and Michael Huebler
Department of Congenital Cardiovascular Surgery, University Children's Hospital, Zurich, Switzerland

Sylvain Choquet
Service d'Hématologie Clinique, Hôpital de la Pitié-Salpêtrière, Paris, France

Ulises López-Cardoza, Carles Díez-López and José González-Costello
Advanced Heart Failure and Transplant Unit, Heart Disease Institute, Hospital Universitari de Bellvitge, IDIBELL, L'Hospitalet de Llobregat, Barcelona, Spain

Robert JH Miller and Kiran Khush
Department of Medicine, Stanford University, Division of Cardiovascular Medicine, Palo Alto, California, United States

Umit Kervan and Dogan Emre Sert
Department of Cardiovascular Surgery, Turkey Yuksek Ihtisas Hospital, Ankara, Turkey

Nesrin Turan
Department of Pathology, Turkey Yuksek Ihtisas Hospital, Ankara, Turkey

Ahmet Dolapoglu
Balikesir Ataturk State Hospital, Cardiovascular Surgery Clinic, Balikesir, Turkey

Eyup Avci
Balikesir University Faculty of Medicine, Cardiology Department, Balikesir, Turkey

Ahmet Celik
Mersin University Faculty of Medicine, Cardiology Department, Mersin, Turkey

Michael Mazzei
Department of General Surgery, Temple University Hospital, USA

Suresh Keshavamurthy, Abul Kashem and Yoshiya Toyoda
Department of Cardiovascular Surgery, Temple University Hospital, USA

Crystal L. Valadon, Erin M. Schumer and Mark S. Slaughter
Department of Cardiovascular and Thoracic Surgery, University of Louisville, Kentucky, USA

Sofia Martin-Suarez, Marianna Berardi, Daniela Votano, Antonio Loforte and Giuseppe Marinelli
Cardiac Surgery Department, S. Orsola-Malpighi Hospital, Bologna University, Bologna, Italy

Luciano Potena and Francesco Grigioni
Cardiology Department, S. Orsola-Malpighi Hospital, Bologna University, Bologna, Italy

Lucas Barbieri and Noedir Stolf
FMUSP-Incor, hospital BP, São Paulo, Brasil

Mariane Manso
FMABC, Santo André, São Paulo, Brasil

Wallace André Pedro da Silva
Hospital Geral de Palmas, Palmas, Brasil

Massimo Baiocchi, Maria Benedetto, Marta Agulli and Guido Frascaroli
Anaesthesiology and Intensive Care Unit, Cardiothoracic and vascular Department, Policlinico S. Orsola University Hospital, Bologna, Italy

Index

www.ingramcontent.com/pod-product-compliance
Lightning Source LLC
Chambersburg PA
CBHW062007190326
41458CB00009B/2992

* 9 7 8 1 6 3 2 4 1 5 6 1 5 *